NEUROPATHY
REVERSED

A HOLISTIC APPROACH
TO ENDING NERVE PAIN

DR. THOMAS A. CHANEY
DR. STEPHANIE J. CHANEY

ISBN: 978-0-9854157-2-3

Important Information for the Reader

This information presented in this book has been compiled from my clinical experience and research. It is offered as a view of the relationship between diet, exercise, emotions, and health. This book is not intended for self-diagnosis or treatment of disease, nor is it a substitute for the advice and care of a licensed health care provider. Sharing of the information in this book with the attending physician is highly desirable.

This book is intended solely to help you make better judgements concerning your long-term health goals. If you are experiencing health problems, you should consult a qualified physician immediately. Remember early examination and detection are important to successful treatment of all diseases.

TABLE OF CONTENTS

PROLOGUE

7:47 am

Thirteen more minutes. Just thirteen minutes before the office switchboard opens. Thirteen minutes until I call my boss to say I can't work today...again. He was so angry the last time. I was sure he was going to fire me right there and then. He is sure to do it this time.

I am out of sick leave, out of vacation days. Another day docked from my paycheck.

What if he really fires me this time! I'll lose my income, lose my health insurance! Oh, how will I manage to pay for all these prescriptions without insurance?

I tried, I really tried to remember – high steps – lift my feet high with each step to prevent tripping over my dropped foot. I have been so good. I haven't tripped for weeks. I'm so tired. All night in the ER, my arm in a cast, unable to work the only job I could find that allowed me to sit all day.

These darn feet! Always failing me, always reminding me of their presence by pinging pain signals all day and all night. I feel like my body has forsaken me. I no longer have control over it.

The simple act of walking, that's it, just to be able to walk without pain, without tripping.

Look at this place. I'm hosting book club tomorrow. The only activity I haven't had to drop. All I have to do is plop my butt down and read. No walking, no standing required. Tonight I'm supposed to clean and bake brownies. How can I do this? Do I cancel? Do I drop out altogether?

What am I going to do?

I'm so tired. Constant, nagging, neuropathy. The doctors have been no help. They just want to write a new prescription and send me out the door. I have tried every pill, every cream, they push on me. Nothing works. Now this. A broken arm.

How did I get here?

8:00 am

CHAPTER 1

AN INTRODUCTION

Our nerves play a crucial role in the body's ability to communicate with its physical environment. They act as pathways through which signals travel from the brain to various organs and tissues. These signals allow us to move, feel sensations, manage our balance, and stand or walk correctly. When the nerves become damaged, their ability to transmit these important signals is disrupted. This can lead to unusual sensations like tingling, numbness, or shooting pains in various parts of the body.

As you can glean from the prologue to this book, neuropathy can be a daily challenge.

If you picked up this book, either you, or a loved one, is living with neuropathy. We want you to know that while neuropathy is challenging, there is hope. With proper treatment and management, dedication, and a positive mindset, anyone with neuropathy can lead a fulfilling and active life.

About Us

We have an integrative health clinic in the Northeast, USA. Through years of clinical practice and continuing education, we have been able to develop healthcare strategies that are effective and impactful. With the rising number of diabetes cases we were seeing, we decided to write Defeat Diabetes: 33 Effective Strategies to End Diabetes – Before it Ends You (published 2017). The book brought us even more patients with diabetes. In the influx of diabetes patients, we saw a high rate of neuropathy as a main clinical complaint. This led us to write a book specific to neuropathy.

Why Choose a Natural Approach for Managing Neuropathy

Many patients with neuropathy are traditionally prescribed various medications, as a means to try managing their symptoms. The medication is intended to reduce pain and numbness and relieve other neuropathy-related symptoms. However, the common medications typically used to treat neuropathy include antidepressants, anticonvulsants, opioids, muscle relaxants, and topical creams, which all come with a wide array of severe and debilitating side-effects. Yet none offers any remedy to end neuropathy. The problems with these commonly prescribed medications are listed in the fine print of the drug inserts, here we have written them plainly.

Antidepressants

Antidepressants alter the way certain chemicals in the brain communicate with one another. Antidepressants like amitriptyline or duloxetine theoretically work by increasing levels of serotonin and norepinephrine in the brain, which is proposed to help reduce pain signals sent from nerves throughout the body. While antidepressants are promoted as "highly effective" in reducing the pain associated with neuropathy, they also come with potential and very severe side-effects. Some antidepressants carry a label warning against depression, weight gain and even suicidal thoughts. Additionally, an article released by *Psychology Today* July 24, 2022, stated that an exhaustive umbrella review of 2022, by Joanna Moncrieff of the University College London and colleagues, found that mental illness is not caused by a chemical imbalance of the brain, which antidepressants claim to "cure."

Anticonvulsants

Anticonvulsant medications, like gabapentin or pregabalin, are thought to reduce nerve-related pain sensations, and the sensation of other symptoms such as tingling or numbness. These drugs work by decreasing abnormal electrical activity in the brain, that trigger painful sensations throughout the body in a neuropathic patient. However, like antidepressants, anticonvulsant medications come with severe side-effects, the lesser of which are dizziness or fatigue. The more major side-effects include conditions such as memory loss, abdominal pain, anxiety, or mood change. And again, these do not remedy the condition of neuropathy.

Opioids

Opioid medications, like oxycodone or morphine, are sometimes prescribed for severe cases of neuropathic pain when other traditional treatments have been unsuccessful. These drugs work by binding to certain opioid receptors in the brain and spinal cord, which can help block pain signals from reaching the rest of the body. However, opioids renowned for a high risk of addiction and other serious side-effects like respiratory depression or constipation. Because of these risks, opioids should only be prescribed under close medical supervision and for very short periods.

Muscle Relaxants

Muscle relaxant medications, like baclofen or tizanidine, are sometimes used to treat muscle spasms or cramping associated with neuropathy. These drugs work by blocking certain signals in the central nervous system, which contribute to muscle tension. While muscle relaxants can be helpful in reducing painful muscle spasms associated with neuropathy, they also come with potential side-effects like drowsiness or dizziness. The more severe of which are nervousness, agitation, headaches, and decreased blood pressure.

Topical Creams

Topical creams containing lidocaine or capsaicin are sometimes also used as an alternative treatment option for neuropathic pain, as they can be applied directly to affected areas on the skin for localized pain relief. Lidocaine works by numbing the nerve endings on the skin's surface, while capsaicin works by desensitizing the nerve fibers over time. While topical creams can be effective in reducing local pain associated with neuropathy, they also come with potential side-effects like skin irritation or burning sensations at the application site.

Other Medications

Additionally, over-the-counter nonsteroidal anti-inflammatory drugs (NSAIDs), such as ibuprofen or naproxen sodium, may traditionally be recommended as treatment. NSAIDs are not typically the first line of treatment for neuropathy, and may only be recommended by some doctors, in certain cases. NSAIDs work by blocking the production of prostaglandins, which are chemicals in the body that cause inflammation and pain. By reducing inflammation and pain signals, NSAIDs may alleviate some of the symptoms associated with neuropathy. It is also worth noting that while NSAIDs can provide relief from nerve pain caused by inflammation, they may not be effective for all types of neuropathies. Some of the side-effects of prolonged use of NSAIDs are stomach ulcers, allergic reactions, indigestion, and, in severe cases, kidney or heart failure.

While medication is a traditional treatment offered to manage neuropathic symptoms, it is important to keep in mind that these medications often have serious side-effects, and do not offer any means of treating the condition of neuropathy itself.

Other more general side-effects of many of these medications include:

- Nausea and vomiting
- Dizziness and lightheadedness
- Fatigue
- Weight gain
- Mood changes
- Constipation
- Dry mouth
- Blurred vision
- Skin rash
- Impaired kidney function

This does not sound like a solution to neuropathy! Mainstream medicine, or medicine driven by health insurance and pharmaceutical companies are neither equipped, nor incentivized, to properly manage diabetes, or neuropathy, let alone patients who have both disorders. So, what are sufferers to do? Look outside the pillbox, find a better way to be effectively treated.

By taking a natural approach to managing neuropathy, you can live without many of these medications. We can teach you which lifestyle choices can help you ease neuropathic pain, enjoy full function of your limbs, and regain a higher quality of life. This book provides you with the information; you choose what is right for you.

> I came to Living Health after being diagnosed with peripheral neuropathy and had already lost feeling in my feet and lower legs. Doctors prescribed Gabapentin and the research was very scary. I found Drs Chaney and took the chance. I now have 98% of my feeling returned, have lost 30 lbs., I am sleeping and eating better, and I have more energy and better focus.
>
> ~ Linda L

The Format of the Book

Although diabetes is the most common cause of neuropathy in the US, there are other causes of neuropathy and as such, this book can help many sufferers regardless of the trigger that brought on neuropathy. Our goal is to provide you with a comprehensive understanding of what living with neuropathy may entail. After reading this book, we hope that you are more equipped to make an informed decision about your care, or better able to both understand the pains and help a loved one who is struggling with this disorder.

Chapter 2 will give you a complete overview of neuropathy including its causes, symptoms, complications, and classifications. This is your foundational chapter that will help you understand later parts of the book. Think of Chapter 2 as the book's nerve center.

Chapter 3 covers the common triggers of diabetic neuropathy. This chapter gives you an understanding of the mechanisms involved in developing neuropathy from different angles. Yes, these are common links for diabetic neuropathy, however, they may also contribute to non-diabetic onset neuropathies.

Chapter 4 provides useful information about food. Knowing what to eat and what to avoid is essential for easing neuropathies. Food is where your new, healthful lifestyle begins.

Chapter 5 entails oxygen. Yes, you will learn how to breathe properly, and you will thank us for it. We also discuss IV ozone for a rapid infusion of oxygen into the bloodstream. Additionally, we cover exercise in this chapter. There are some simple, beginner exercises to get you started until you are ready for the advanced versions noted in the chapter.

Chapter 6 is all about an amazing wellness system called HOCATT. It is an all-in-one machine that provides amazing results. Your body will love it.

Chapter 7 explains red-light therapy and how it can ease neuropathic pain.

Chapter 8 digs into magnet therapy. Your body's magnetic fields can become unbalanced for a variety of reasons. Magnet therapy can help get your magnetism back in balance.

Chapter 9 gets you moving with vibration therapy. With only minutes a day, this therapy can truly wake up your nerves. It is a great sensation.

Chapter 10 There are specific frequencies that can heal parts of the body. We focus on frequencies for regenerating nerves. Frequency therapy really makes you feel energized.

Chapter 11 describes the phases of healing. After reading the previous chapters, we want you to understand the stages a person goes through in the healing process. The lifestyle suggestions and therapies provided in this book are not overnight cures. Thus, it is vital for people embarking on this healing journey to know that it will take time to get there.

Chapter 12 is the conclusion where we wrap things up.

A Future Outlook

With an early diagnosis and treatment, individuals with neuropathy can often manage their symptoms effectively and maintain a high level of function and quality of life. Depending on the severity of the condition and the type and degree of nerve damage, some cases of neuropathy may even be reversed.

It is important for individuals living with neuropathy to seek support from friends, family members or healthcare professionals who understand what they are going through. Support groups for individuals living with chronic pain conditions like neuropathy are also available both online, and in-person. These groups provide opportunities for individuals to connect with others who share similar experiences and may offer an individual dealing with neuropathy the support and understanding they need.

We wish you well on your healing journey.

CHAPTER 2

OVERVIEW OF NEUROPATHY

N europathy is defined as a disease (pathos) of the nerves (neuro). It can be caused by diabetes, other disorders trauma, and even treatment regimens such as chemotherapy. This condition is sometimes termed peripheral neuropathy (PN), due to peripheral rather than central nerve damage.

Damage to the nerves outside the central nervous system (the brain and spinal cord) causes weakness, altered sensation, and numbness in the hands and feet.

It may also impact other parts of the body. PN is not a single health condition, but rather a term to describe a range of health problems stemming from damaged peripheral nerves. People usually describe the pain stemming from PN as a sharp, burning, or tingling sensation.

Living with Neuropathy

The impact of neuropathy on daily activities can vary depending on the severity of the condition. In mild cases, individuals may only experience occasional discomfort or difficulty performing certain tasks. However, in more severe cases, neuropathy can significantly impair mobility and cause significant limitations in daily life.

Similarly, neuropathy can also affect an individual's ability to grip objects properly while cooking or performing other manual tasks. It can be challenging to manage utensils or cookware, due to the decreased sensation in the fingers. In addition to these physical limitations, individuals with neuropathy may also experience fatigue and weakness that further impairs their ability to perform daily activities. They may need more rest breaks throughout the day or require assistance from others when performing certain tasks.

Every step can be a challenge. The sensation of walking on pins and needles or feeling like their feet are numb can make it difficult to maintain proper footing and balance. This can increase the risk of falls and other accidents, which can lead to further injury or complications. Additionally, neuropathy may cause weakness in the legs that may result in difficulty lifting the foot off the ground during each step. This condition is called "foot drop," and often requires individuals to lift their legs higher than usual while walking, to prevent tripping or stumbling.

Moreover, individuals with neuropathy may also experience muscle cramps or spasms that can be painful and make it difficult to walk normally. These symptoms may occur randomly throughout the day or become more frequent during periods of increased activity. Furthermore, neuropathy can affect an individual's gait pattern (the way they walk) causing them to shuffle their feet or take shorter steps than usual. This change in gait pattern may be a compensatory mechanism used by the body to avoid putting too much pressure on areas that are experiencing discomfort or pain.

In addition to the physical symptoms, neuropathy may also take an emotional toll. It is not uncommon for patients with neuropathy to feel anxious or depressed due to the impact of their condition, and they may become very frustrated by their inability to do things they once easily enjoyed. Thus, it can be a real struggle to remain positive in the face of ongoing challenges.

Moreover, living with a chronic condition like neuropathy can also lead to social isolation and feelings of loneliness. Individuals may feel they do not want to be a burden to others with their struggles or worry that they will be judged for not being able to do things that others take for granted. The financial burden associated with neuropathy treatments can also contribute to increased emotional stress when living with this condition. The cost of medication, doctor's visits, and other medical expenses can quickly add up.

These factors contribute to increased stress levels and negatively impact an individual's mental health, on top of the physical disabilities. Any healthcare professional who works closely with patients living with neuropathy understands how challenging this condition can be. That is why it is important for patients to seek proper care from healthcare and mental health professionals who specialize in treating this condition.

The Sensations of Neuropathic Pain

Neuropathy can be a difficult pain to understand for those who have not experienced it themselves. An individual with neuropathic pain may not show any obvious conditions that could warrant such pain, like a wound or signs of severe damage. However, neuropathic pain can be very debilitating and excruciating. Pain of this type is tied in the various forms of "over stimulated" nerves. Neuropathic pain is often characterized by sensations such as "burning," tingling, shooting, "stabbing," or electric shock-like pains. They can be constant or intermittent and vary in intensity from person to person. For those dealing with neuropathy-related pains, these sensations can be mildly annoying, to severely debilitating. Examples can be a patient with a constant "buzzing" in their hands, to the patient who felt as though they were being burned when their nightgown brushed against their skin.

<u>Burning</u>

The most common symptom of neuropathic pain is "burning." The nerve fibers have become overactive and send false signals, which create a burning sensation. The patient literally feels as though their skin is on fire. The burning sensation of neuropathic pain is thought to be caused by damaged nerves that are no longer able to effectively transmit signals from the body to the brain and are "hyperactive," often shooting off signals that do not match the level of sensation from the actual environment (as with the nightgown). Even a light touch can cause the nerve fibers to "misfire" and create a burning pain.

Tingling and numbness

Tingling ("pins-and-needles") and numbness are common sensations of neuropathy. Tingling may also feel like a "buzzing," "prickling," or a "crawling sensation," as if insects were crawling on the skin. Numbness refers to a lack of feeling or sensation in an affected area. This can make it difficult for individuals to perform everyday tasks, such as holding objects or walking without tripping over themselves. These sensations occur due to damage or dysfunctions of the nerves, which can disrupt the ability to communicate effectively with the brain. The hands and feet are particularly susceptible to tingling and numbing sensations, as they contain a high number of nerve endings. Many common causes of this type of sensation are nerve damage related to chronic conditions, such as diabetes, autoimmune disorders, and infections such as Lyme disease, exposure to toxins (like chemotherapy drugs and statin drugs), or physical trauma such as car accidents.

Shooting Pains

Shooting pains are a common symptom of nerve damage that can occur anywhere on the skin. These pains are caused by damaged nerve endings that send incorrect signals to the brain, leading to intense and sometimes debilitating pain. These pains can last for seconds, or minutes at a time. The causes of nerve damage such as this vary, but may stem from conditions such as diabetes, autoimmune disorders, infections (like shingles or Lyme disease), exposure to toxins (like chemotherapy drugs or statins), or physical trauma, like as car accidents.

Stabbing Pains

Stabbing sensations are a common symptom of neuropathy. These sensations may feel intense jolts through the body, or sudden sharp pains in a specific area without any warning. They can occur anywhere on the body but are most commonly felt in the hands and feet.

"Electric Shocks"

The exact mechanisms behind these "electric shock" sensations of neuropathy are still not fully understood. However, it is believed that the nerve damage disrupts the normal flow of electrical impulses along the nerve fibers. This may lead to erratic signaling patterns that result in abnormal sensations, like electric shocks.

The severity and frequency of these varied symptoms can vary widely between individuals depending on factors such as age, underlying health conditions, and lifestyle habits.

Symptoms of Neuropathy

There are some early signs which could indicate the onset of neuropathy. It is valuable to know what some of them are so you can seek care from your healthcare provider. Below are some of the common symptoms of neuropathy.

Paresthesia

One symptom that is commonly associated with neuropathy is a tingling sensation in the feet and hands, otherwise known as paresthesia. This sensation may start as mild and become more intense, as time goes on. It may also feel like a prickling, burning, numbing, or even itching. This symptom can progress to the point of extreme pain and, if left untreated, could become debilitating.

Muscle Weakness

Muscle weakness can cause difficulties with everyday tasks, such as walking or getting dressed. Muscle weakness can lead to falls. You may notice that you are unable to stand for long periods without becoming fatigued, or that your balance has become compromised.

Sensory Issues

Sensory issues are another common symptom associated with neuropathy. Some people experience decreased sensitivity in their hands and feet, while others have an increased sensitivity, both of which can make everyday activities (like putting on socks or shoes) very uncomfortable. Many times, these issues may cause significant discomfort when standing or walking. Other sensory disturbances may include a loss or reduction of sensation such as temperature changes and touch sensitivity. Hypersensitivity may also be the case, where a person feels an increased sensitivity to touch, sound, light, or other stimuli. The individual experiences an exaggerated response to these normal stimuli, often describing them as feeling "intensely uncomfortable."

Loss of Reflexes

The loss of reflexes is often overlooked. The "Achilles reflex," which is checked by tapping the calf with a hammer and measuring the response of the foot, is one example. This reflex should cause an obvious jerk or movement of the foot, when tapped. Other reflexes like the biceps, triceps, patellar and plantar responses may also be impaired in individuals with neuropathy.

Pain

Burning or stabbing pains in the feet and hands are common symptoms in those who suffer from neuropathy, and if left untreated can become debilitating over time. Here, chiropractic treatment can be of great relief. Some chiropractors have specialized in treating neuropathy-related pain through a variety of techniques such as soft tissue massage, laser therapy, and spinal adjustments.

Changes in Skin and Nails

Changes in the skin can be seen in the form of dryness or a discoloration of the skin, while changes in nails can be seen as a thickening of the nails. Additionally, this can lead to poor wound healing with cuts or injuries that would normally not be an issue. In severe cases, it can even lead to ulcers developing on your feet or hands that do not heal properly, especially in the case of diabetic neuropathy.

Weakness of Arms and Legs

Another symptom that may be an indication of neuropathy is "a feeling of weakness" in the arms or legs. This can be mild or severe, depending on the severity of the condition. Sometimes, this symptom goes together with muscle atrophy, which results in a decrease of the muscle mass in those areas. The individual may also have trouble with coordination and balance, leading to falls or other accidents.

Sleep Disturbance

One of the most common ways that neuropathy affects sleep is through pain and discomfort. Individuals with neuropathy may experience chronic pain, tingling, or burning sensations that make it difficult to fall asleep or stay asleep throughout the night. Lack of quality sleep can compound the physical and emotional symptoms of neuropathy.

In addition to pain and discomfort, neuropathy can also cause changes in the breathing pattern during sleep. This is due to a certain nerve damage which affects the muscles involved in breathing, leading to conditions like sleep apnea where breathing stops and starts repeatedly throughout the night. Sleep apnea can further disrupt normal sleep patterns and leave individuals feeling tired and groggy during the day.

Additionally, neuropathy may further affect the levels of neurotransmitters, like serotonin and melatonin, which regulate moods and promote healthy sleep. When nerve damage interferes with these neurotransmitter systems, it can lead to insomnia or other sleep disorders that can make it difficult for individuals with neuropathy to get adequate rest.

If you experience any of the above symptoms, it is important to speak with your healthcare professional about the possibility of neuropathy. Neuropathy can be a difficult condition with which to live, but it does not have to control your entire life. By understanding the signs and symptoms of neuropathy, you may be able to take the necessary steps toward getting proper treatment and management of your condition. With the right support system and the care of experienced professionals, living with neuropathy can be made easier. An early diagnosis can mean more effective treatments and better outcomes!

Potential Complications

Neuropathy is a progressive condition and, if left untreated, it can lead to several other complications detrimental to an individual's health and quality of life.

Foot Ulcers

One of the most common complications associated with peripheral neuropathy is foot ulcers. Foot ulcers occur when pressure sores form on the feet, usually when an area of skin is repeatedly rubbed or pressed against. These sores are particularly vulnerable to infection, and if not treated adequately can develop into serious infections such as cellulitis or sepsis. When nerve damage occurs, the body's normal sensation decreases, meaning that people do not as easily feel pain in their feet. This is typically very common in diabetic neuropathy.

Increased Risks of Falls

Neuropathy can lead to falls which are especially dangerous if the patient already has weak bones and low muscle strength, due to age or other poor health conditions. As nerve damage occurs, the muscles in the feet become weakened. As a result, people are more likely to suffer from issues with their balance, which can then lead to falls. The individual may experience an "abnormal" sensation in their feet, which can cause them to stumble or become unsteady. They may also have decreased reflexes, making it difficult for them to respond quickly to sudden movements.

Charcot Foot Deformity

Charcot Foot Deformity is a condition where the joints and bones of the foot become weakened. This can lead to painful deformities and an inability to walk properly, which puts the person at risk of further complications, such as infections. A gradual change in the shape of the feet or ankles develop, creating a "hammertoe" or "arch collapse." Here, traditional treatment is often in the form of surgery, casting, orthotics, and physical therapy.

For this reason, it is essential to have regular check-ups with your medical practitioner if you are suffering from neuropathy. By catching and managing any potential complications early on, you can prevent them from getting worse. Your practitioner may also suggest certain lifestyle changes, such as quitting smoking and controlling your blood sugar levels if you have diabetes, to help slow the progression of neuropathy and lower the risk of other complications.

Taking care of your feet with regular check-ups and proper foot care is essential for managing neuropathy. If you happen to notice any changes or feel any pain in your feet, seek medical advice immediately. With good management, many of the potential complications associated with neuropathy can be avoided.

There Are Four Types of Diabetic Neuropathy

Not every neuropathy is "one size fits all." We know how that phrase does not work for most things. Neuropathy is no exception.

Peripheral Neuropathy

Peripheral neuropathy (PN) goes by various names: peripheral diabetic nerve pain and distal polyneuropathy. PN is the most common form of neuropathy caused by diabetes. It affects the nerves leading to your extremities, such as your feet, legs, hands, and arms. The nerves going to your feet are the longest in your body. They can be more than 6 feet (1.8 meters) in adults. Nerves reaching the feet literally stretch from head to toe! Because the nerves leading to your feet are so long, it is most often these nerves that get damaged; simply because there are more of them to be damaged. The nerves in your feet depend on blood vessels to feed them. The further away from the heart, the smaller the vessel. Because they are small, they become clogged first and more frequently. This blockage stops the flow of oxygen and nutrients to the nerves. For nerves to be healthy, they need oxygen and nutrients. This type of nerve damage can lead to the foot problems often associated with diabetes, including foot deformities, infections, ulcers, and amputations.

Proximal Neuropathy

Proximal neuropathy can also be called diabetic amyotrophy. The "myo" in the word means "muscle," so this is a form of neuropathy that can cause muscle weakness. It specifically affects the muscles in the upper part of your legs, buttocks, and hips. Proximal neuropathy is the second most common type of diabetic neuropathy. It usually affects older adults with diabetes and, as opposed to peripheral neuropathy, it usually resolves over time, or with treatment.

Autonomic Neuropathy

Autonomic nerves are supposed to keep your body running as it should. Many functions happen in your body without you consciously thinking about them; your heart pumps, you breathe, and your stomach digests food. The autonomic nervous system controls those actions. The autonomic nervous system should maintain your body's homeostasis, which would be its normal, balanced state. Autonomic neuropathy can seem daunting because it can affect so many of your body's systems, from your digestive tract to how well you can see. However, remember that your symptoms depend on what specific nerves in the autonomic nervous system are damaged.

<u>Focal Neuropathy</u>

All the types of diabetic neuropathy mentioned above, peripheral, autonomic, and proximal, are examples of polyneuropathy. "Poly" means that they affect several nerves. Focal neuropathy, also called mononeuropathy, by contrast, affects a specific nerve. Focal neuropathy, which comes on suddenly, most often affects nerves in the head (especially ones that go to the eyes) but can also affect the torso and legs, causing stabbing pain, numbness, and weakness. Symptoms tend to resolve within 6 to 8 weeks; however, they can remain chronic in individuals with diabetes. People with diabetes are at higher risk for developing focal neuropathy.

Causes of Nerve Damage

Peripheral neuropathy is nerve damage produced by various diseases rather than a single illness. A myriad of health conditions can cause PN. In neuropathy, nerve signaling is interrupted in three ways:

- Loss of normal signal functions,
- Sending of inappropriate signals without any impulse,
- Distortions to the signals being transmitted.

Unlike nerve cells in the central nervous system, peripheral nerve cells continue to develop throughout life. Symptoms may range from moderate to severe. The type of nerve fibers damaged, and the type and intensity of injury, determine these symptoms. Symptoms might appear for days, weeks, or years.

Diabetes is the most common cause of PN. Other causes include trauma-related, HIV-related, chemotherapy-related, and autoimmune-related diseases. Autoimmune disorders are conditions in which the immune system attacks self-tissues or organs. Examples of autoimmune disorders include type-2 diabetes, Celiac disease, Alzheimer's disease, and arthritis. Disorders known to be associated with PN include Sjogren's disease, systemic lupus erythematosis, rheumatoid arthritis, Guillain-Barré syndrome, chronic inflammatory demyelinating polyneuropathy, and vasculitis.

What Role Does Diabetes Play in Causing Neuropathy?

Nerve issues can occur at any time within a person struggling with diabetes. In some cases, neuropathy is the first indication of diabetes. Significant nerve issues (clinical neuropathy) might occur during the first ten years after a diagnosis. The longer a person has diabetes, the more likely a neuropathic condition will develop.

Although the specific causes of diabetic neuropathy are unknown, several variables may play a role in developing the condition, such as:

- High Blood Sugar. High blood glucose damages neurons by causing chemical changes which impede their capacity to send impulses. It can also harm the blood arteries which supply the neurons with oxygen and nourishment.
- Metabolic Factors. High triglyceride, cholesterol, and glucose levels are linked to an increased risk of neuropathy. Neuropathy is more likely to manifest itself in people who are overweight or obese.
- Genetic Factors. Some hereditary characteristics may predispose some people to nerve illnesses more than others.

A staggering 45% of patients with type-2 diabetes and 54% of those with type-1 diabetes develop some form of neuropathy.(Hicks and Selvin) Hicks and Selvin also state that depending on age, years of diabetes and type of diabetes, up to 51% of diabetics suffer from peripheral neuropathy. At the time of a diabetic diagnosis, neuropathy is predicted to already be present in 7.5% of patients. Distal symmetric polyneuropathy accounts for more than half of all cases. The rest comprises focal syndromes, such as carpal tunnel syndrome (14-30%), radiculopathies/plexopathies, and cranial neuropathies. As many people with the condition are asymptomatic at first, diagnosis relies heavily on a thorough neurological examination by a primary care physician. Additional diagnostic methods, such as autonomic or quantitative sensory testing, might lead to a more significant number being documented in time.

Prevalence of Peripheral Neuropathy in the United States

To acquire a clearer picture of the peripheral neuropathy prevalence in the US, let us categorize incidents according to cause.

Diabetic Peripheral Neuropathy

Peripheral neuropathy affects 28% of individuals with diabetes in the United States. The diagnosis of diabetic PN is based on both clinical indicators and quantitative tests. It may exist despite the absence of symptoms. Prevalence of diabetic PN in type-1 diabetes mellitus is 28.70% and in type-2 diabetes mellitus it is 50.70%.

The risk for painful neuropathy is increased in type-2 diabetes, women, and those of South Asian ethnicity.(Feldman *et al.*)

Profound consequences can come with diabetic PN. Diabetes mellitus significantly increases the risk of lower limb amputation, with around 50% of people with diabetes developing a foot ulcer over their lifespan. Furthermore, neuropathic pain and reduced sensations can lead to various negative consequences, including falls, a lowered quality of life, limitations in daily activities, and signs of depression.

HIV-Associated Sensory Peripheral Neuropathy

The most frequent neurological consequence of HIV infection is PN. This illness, which has a detrimental influence on HIV/AIDS patients, comes in various clinical forms. The most prevalent kind of HIV neuropathy is sensory neuropathy (HIV-SN), which affects up to two-thirds of individuals. Primary HIV-associated distal sensory polyneuropathy (HIV-DSP) and ART toxic neuropathy (ATN) are the two primary forms of HIV-associated distal sensory peripheral neuropathies, afflicting 30 – 67% of individuals with advanced HIV.

Postherpetic Neuralgia (PHN)

PHN is a form of neuropathy caused by the reactivation of the herpes zoster virus. The virus persists in an inactive state within the sensory ganglion of the spinal cord until the patient's immunocompetence deteriorates due to aging, HIV infection, cancer, or immunosuppressive treatments, at which point it can reactivate. According to data from Clinical Infectious Diseases, the total incident rate of PHN was 57.5 cases per 100,000 people a year. In addition, researchers also discovered that the proportion of people with herpes zoster who acquired PHN increased between 2007 and 2018, compared to 1994 to 2006.

Chemotherapy-Induced Peripheral Neuropathy

Chemotherapy-induced peripheral neuropathy is the most prevalent complication of neurological cancer therapy. It is a chemotherapy-related side effect that is dose-dependent. Chemotherapy drugs damage the sensory nerves in the posterior ganglion of the spinal cord. Approximately one-third of cancer patients are given chemotherapy. Most individuals starting chemotherapy develop symptoms within six months. As the treatment continues, the symptoms may increase. In many situations, once the therapy is stopped, improvement is seen.

Guillain-Barré Syndrome (GBS)

GBS incidents are low (although connected to roughly half of multiple sclerosis cases), however, the cumulative effect of lifelong impairment in young people constitutes a significant public health issue. The illness can strike anyone at any age, from infancy to the golden years. There is a linear increase in incidents with aging as a decrease in immune suppressor systems develops, which causes an increased vulnerability to autoimmune illnesses.

Chronic Inflammatory Demyelinating Polyneuropathy (CIDP)

CIDP has relatively limited epidemiological data. It is a rare illness, and the neurophysiological and nerve biopsy tests needed to detect it are complex. Thus, it is likely underdiagnosed. There are currently no accurate population estimates of its prevalence. However, Broers reported a prevalence of CIDP ranging from 0.7 to 10.3 cases per 100,000 people.

Carpal Tunnel Syndrome

Carpal tunnel occurs due to compression on the median nerve, traveling through the wrist's transverse carpal ligament. It effects women more than men and is a prevalent diagnosis in outpatient neurology and rheumatology clinics. Still, there needs to be more information regarding its prevalence in the general population. There are several risk factors for developing carpal tunnel syndrome. Highest risk factors occur in persons with repetitive wrist motions, such as some line-factory positions, and high-force hammering. Other known risk factors are comprised of heredity, pregnancy, hemodialysis, wrist facture and/or dislocation, hand/wrist deformity, arthritic disorders including gout, hypothyroidism, hormone imbalance, diabetes, alcoholism, amyloid deposits, older age, and tumor in the carpal tunnel.

Alcohol Consumption

People who abuse alcohol are more likely to develop peripheral nerve damage. Whether this is due to a direct toxic impact from alcohol, or a chronic nutritional deficit has been debated for a long time. It is believed in the United States that 25% to 66% of chronic alcoholics suffer from neuropathy. However, the prevalence in the general population is unclear. The bulk of the patients are middle-class working males, and those who drink continuously are more impacted than those who drink sporadically.

Traditional Avenues Related to Treatment of Neuropathy

Various therapies are available to assist in alleviating symptoms and peripheral neuropathy. The phrase "traditional/conventional neuropathy therapy" refers to treatment methods doctors have used for a long time. Etiology determines the type of treatment for peripheral neuropathy. Some of the most frequent therapies are physical therapy, surgery, and injections for increased nerve pressure. Approaches can be pharmacological and non-pharmacological.

Medical Management of Pain

Headaches, stomach discomfort, ulcers, dizziness, and elevated blood pressure, are all possible side effects. Over- the-counter, non-steroidal, anti-inflammatory medicines like ibuprofen and aspirin are examples of this regimen. These medicines can assist with managing pain, and more potent medications (such as antidepressants or anticonvulsants) are sometimes also administered to handle the pain. None of these medications, however, treat the actual condition of neuropathy.

Neuropathic pain is a complex condition to manage. It can be weakened and managed by various painkillers and antiseizure medications. In many patients, current treatment techniques fail to provide adequate or tolerable pain relief and come with unwanted side-effects. The primary reasons why conventional therapies for neuropathic pain management fail can be summarized into four categories:

1. Inadequate diagnosis and a lack of knowledge of the disease processes involved.
2. Poor care of associated disorders.
3. Misunderstanding or selection of treatment choices.
4. Use of unsuitable measurements for evaluating the condition.

Clomipramine and amitriptyline have been proven to function better for neuropathy than the newer selective serotonin reuptake inhibitors (SSRIs). While SSRIs are claimed by some to be more successful in treating depression, they have less of an effect on neuropathy. Prozac®, Zoloft®, Cymbalta®, Celexa®, and Nardil® are some of the most well-known brands. However, dry mouth, headaches, sexual dysfunction, even suicidal tendencies, are all known adverse effects.

Gralise™, Neuraptine™ and Lyrica® are brand names of the most often prescribed anticonvulsants. Patients using these drugs, which include Gabapentin and tiagabine, have experienced less discomfort. Dizziness, tiredness, nausea, memory loss, sleepiness, and weight gain are some of the unwanted side effects.

Narcotic medications reduce neuronal excitability (which causes pain) by binding to specific receptors in the brain and the peripheral nervous system. Codeine, hydrocodone, morphine, and oxycodone are common examples. Nausea, vomiting, and constipation are common and known adverse effects.

Surgical Treatment

For some kinds of neuropathies, surgery is a commonly used approach. Nerve roots, compressed by protruding disks ("pinched nerves") in the back or neck, are often treated surgically. Surgical procedures can release the afflicted nerve root and allow it to recover.

Neurosurgical decompression is frequently used to treat facial trigeminal neuralgia. Mononeuropathy caused by compression, trapping, or, in rare cases, tumors, or infections, may necessitate surgery to relieve nerve compression. Surgery does not assist polyneuropathies with more widespread nerve degeneration, such as diabetic neuropathy.

Surgery or interventional treatments which seek to relieve pain by cutting or damaging nerves are usually ineffective as they worsen nerve injury. The portions of the peripheral and central nervous systems above the incision frequently keep sending pain signals (phantom pain). These surgeries have mostly been superseded by more advanced and less harmful treatments, such as electrically stimulating remaining peripheral nerve fibers or pain-processing regions of the spinal cord or brain.

Other Approaches for Treatment of Neuropathy

Alternative therapies are also available to people who want to do more than the convention therapies alone, for those who have not had good outcomes with conventional treatments and for those who prefer to address neuropathy through less invasive, non-pharmaceutical ways.

Acupuncture

An ancient practice, acupuncture involves the insertion of fine needles into various points on the body. Acupuncture can both stimulate nerve pathways, and optimize blood flow, which allows vital nutrients to reach damaged nerves. Acupuncture therapy may take several sessions before realizing results.

Alpha-Lipoic Acid

Oxidative stress contributes to nerve damage. People with diabetes are at higher risk for oxidative stress. Acute infusion of alpha-lipoic acid improves microcirculation in patients with diabetic neuropathy. Supplementation with alpha-lipoic acid can affect blood sugar levels, upset the stomach and cause skin rashes. Always consult your doctor before implementing a supplement protocol.

Amino Acids

Non-essential amino acids, such as acetyl-L-carnitine and serine, possess antioxidant properties, can slow down nerve damage, and may ease pain associated with neuropathy. Amino acids might benefit people who have undergone chemotherapy and people with diabetes. Side effects include nausea and vomiting.

Medicinal Herbs

There is a long list of herbs that may be used for treating neuropathic pain. A short list includes:

- Artemisia
- Curcuma longa
- Ginkgo biloba
- Saffron
- Sage

These herbs have anti-inflammatory, antioxidant, neuro-protective properties. For a comprehensive review of medicinal herbs used to treat neuropathic pain, see Forouzanfar and Hosseinzadeh. Before implementing a supplement protocol, always check with your doctor first as some herbs interact with medications.

Spinal Cord Stimulation (SCS)

SCS is a type of pain neuromodulation. SCS for the treatment of refractory painful diabetic peripheral neuropathy showed a substantial decrease in pain intensity ratings, which lasted at least six months.

Transcutaneous Electrical Nerve Stimulation (TENS)

TENS is a non-invasive pain treatment technique that may be utilized for various ailments. The treatment involves placing electrodes on the skin, at the location of pain or near related nerves and then providing a mild electrical current. Several studies have demonstrated TENS to alleviate neuropathic symptoms linked with diabetes.

Our Approaches for Treatment of Neuropathy

Our approaches involve lifestyle changes for long-lasting results, without the need for life-long medications, supplements, or pain.

> *The care at Living Health is personal and professional, knowledgeable, and caring. I've experienced improvement in my diabetes, weight, and neuropathy that I hadn't known were possible.*
>
> *~ Linda P*

Dietary Lifestyle

No, we do not put you on a diet, rather we teach you about food. Food can be harmful, healing or neutral. We first want you to heal, then consume both healing and neutral foods. You will learn which foods are harmful and thus, know what to avoid in order to have better health.

Increased Oxygenation

By simple breathing techniques, hyperbaric chambers, and ozone therapy, the increase of oxygen to the bloodstream optimizes blood flow, which is necessary for rebuilding nerves.

Exercise

Although many of the most frequent causes of peripheral neuropathy are incurable, it is essential to recognize that regular exercise cannot only help avoid some of them but has also been shown to help relieve some of the most unpleasant symptoms.

Whole Body Stimulation by HOCATT

This novel device stimulates the entire body. HOCATT incorporates a host of therapies, conducted at one time. An HOCATT session saves time, when needing relief from neuropathic symptoms.

Low-Intensity Red Light

In individuals with diabetic peripheral neuropathy, pulsed infrared light treatment (PILT) has improved peripheral sensitivity.

Magnet Therapy

By optimizing your magnetic energy flow, healing of nerves can occur.

Vibration Therapy

Whole-body vibration (WBV) training is a novel form of somatosensory stimulation (SSS) exercise, which has gained popularity in sports training and rehabilitation over the past decade.

Frequency Therapy

Frequencies are all around us. Some are harmful, as felt by some people living or working near cellphone towers, or electrical transmission towers. Other frequencies are healing. Focused, specific frequencies can restore damaged nerves.

Personalizing a combination of these therapies into your unique plan, can help you live a better quality of life.

The Experience of People Seeking Care for Neuropathy

The primary symptoms of peripheral neuropathy are neuromuscular, with physical pain in the feet, hands, arms, back, and knees. Numbness and tingling are the most common complaints.

Furthermore, co-morbid disorders, such as depression, are typical consequences of chronic pain and contribute to patients' everyday impairment and disability.

Clinical and administrative difficulties lead to patients with peripheral neuropathy receiving less-than-optimal treatment. Since the situation is not considered an emergency, the already overburdened personnel often cannot respond quickly and comprehensively. Even though the number of dedicated pain clinics is growing worldwide, only a tiny percentage of patients are referred to pain experts. Harden and Cohen reported that of 703 individuals in the UK with neuropathic pain, the majority (79%) had been in pain for more than a year before receiving a referral to a pain clinic. This delay harms their clinical care and long-term results.

Unfortunately, evidence suggests that treatment of neuropathic pain is frequently insufficient. An explanation for this is that pain perception is influenced by three aspects, psychological, psycho-behavioral, and sociocultural factors. Many neuropathy patients say their pain has affected their emotions, sleep, relationships, and ability to operate.

Though combination treatment is superior to administering a single pharmacological agent, it may not be enough to relieve pain completely. Non- pharmaceutical therapies, such as physiotherapy, counselling, or alternative approaches, may also be necessary. Cognitive behavioral therapy can help people with chronic pain, reduce discomfort and improve positive behavior expression, evaluation, and coping.

Also, relaxation treatments such as progressive muscle relaxation, regulated breathing, and guided visualization may be beneficial.

With a host of different kinds of neuropathies, causes or triggers, and treatment options that span the holistic to conventional medicine approaches, managing neuropathy can be overwhelming. Continue reading for a better understanding of the pathogenesis of neuropathies, environmental triggers or exacerbators of neuropathies and options for alleviating the conditions associated with your specific neuropathy.

CHAPTER 3

LINKS TO DIABETIC NEUROPATHY: SUGAR, INFLAMMATION, STATINS

S ugar may be sweet, but it has a nasty side to it. Everyone knows sugar is detrimental for diabetics, however, the power of sugar's destruction is far-reaching in the form of inflammation and immune suppression for many people who do not have diabetes. Every cell in our bodies uses sugar from our bloodstream for fuel. Too much sugar, however, can lead to diabetes, cancer and, yes, neuropathy.

Brazilian sugarcane was introduced to the Caribbean around 1647 when the industry was established, and sugar refinement in the US began its history. Sugar today is a regular part of many diets in the West. According to the American Heart Association, US adults average 77 grams (roughly 18 teaspoons) of sugar per day. That is three times the recommended daily allowance for women and two times the recommendation for men. In one year, that equals 6570 teaspoons of sugar: over sixty pounds! These numbers may seem exaggerated at first, but if we consider that many types of sugars are often "hidden" in various types of food, such an amount is not surprising at all.

Refined and processed sugar is often found in white sugar (sucrose), corn syrup, and dextrose. These processed and concentrated sugars are often found in breakfast cereals, bread, jams, butter, condiments/sauces, peanut butter, pies, tomato sauce, and a broad range of processed and pre-made meals.

Back in the 19th century, the average sugar intake for one person was just about 5 pounds per year. Sugar consumption levels have continued to increase at alarming rates, with no indication of a reversal. Some research demonstrates that the more sugar someone consumes, the higher the risk of developing health problems later in life.

The Glycemic Index

Every type of food that contains natural or synthetic sugar is measured according to its glycemic index (GI). This index is measured on a scale from 0 to 100, depending on the impact it has on blood glucose levels. Foods that are ranked with a low GI are often deemed healthier and have less of an effect regarding spiking blood sugar levels, while those with a high GI score are considered to have a strong effect on spiking blood sugar levels and can be damaging to our systems.

Here are just some of the healthier benefits of consuming foods with a low GI:

- Decreased levels of cholesterol,
- Lessened risk of developing diabetes,
- Increased energy levels,
- Controlled cravings and hunger episodes,
- Raises sensitivity to insulin,
- More stable body weight and loss of excess fat,
- Lower risk of developing heart diseases.

It is essential to be aware of the GI score of the various foods you eat. Foods with a low GI score release controlled amounts of sugar in a gradual process when digested, compared to foods with a higher GI score. The gradual release of sugar into the bloodstream helps to maintain blood sugar levels more stably, while preventing sudden spikes in blood sugar that can lead to energy crashes throughout the day.

Be aware some low-GI foods can exacerbate diabetes, especially type-2 diabetes, in some individuals. Foods such as seaweed, apricots, lentils, chickpeas (garbanzo beans) peanuts, wheat, zucchini, milk (cow and goat), oats, spinach, and cooked garlic. Dr Kharrazian, *et al.* studied the immune cross-reactivity between low-GI foods and pancreatic tissues. The results were certainly surprising. These foods have similar protein structure to some of the tissues related to diabetes. Thus, for some individuals, consuming these foods will make the diabetic condition worse. If you are consuming only low-GI foods and your diabetes is not improving, consider being tested for IgG food sensitivity (not food allergy).

The "sugar crash," as we know it, is quite common. When consuming foods with high sugar content, the blood sugar levels peak about an hour after eating, only to fall suddenly thereafter. This is the culprit behind sudden energy crashes and tiredness after consuming something with a high sugar content.

The Link Between Sugar and Cholesterol

The key to cholesterol is that there must be a balance between the "good" and the "bad." High-density lipoprotein (HDL) is considered the "good" cholesterol, while Low-density lipoprotein (LDL) is considered the "bad" cholesterol. Lipoproteins carry cholesterol through the peripheral bloodstream. Additionally, triglycerides need to be evaluated in this scenario. Triglycerides are a type of fat (lipid) in your blood. When you eat, your body converts any calories it does not need to use right away into triglycerides. Your doctor will measure these markers when assessing your potential diabetes. Ideally, you want your HDL level to be at least 60, but higher is better, your optimal LDL level would be less than 100 mg/dL and triglyceride level should be less than 150 mg/dL. High triglyceride and LDL levels could increase your risk for heart disease.

If you have, or are suspected of having, diabetes or heart disease, your doctor has already ordered a lipid profile panel on you. The lipid panel measures the amount of cholesterol and other fats circulating in your bloodstream. The lipid profile has served practitioners for years, however, there is a new, FDA-cleared test now available. This new test more accurately assesses risk for cardiovascular disease, stroke, and insulin resistance (the lipid profile cannot assess insulin resistance). See the lipids testing table below for a comparison of the standard test versus the NMR LipoProfile®.

NMR LipoProfile® includes lipid subclasses, average sizes of the particles, and amount of cholesterol inside the lipid particle, this information is a more accurate measurement of risk.

			NMR-LipoProfile®	Lipid Profile
Cardiovascular	Disease	Markers	LDL-P (particle number)	LDL
			LDL-C (cholesterol carried)	HDL
			Triglycerides	Triglycerides (TG)
			Total Cholesterol	Total Cholesterol
			HDL-P	Non-HDL-C
			HDL-C	TG to HDL ratio
Diabetes	Markers		Small LDL-P	
			LDL size	
			LP-IR Score (insulin resistance)	

By assessing particle numbers and sizes, a calculation of risk for cardiovascular disease can be accomplished. By measuring the small LDL particles, an insulin resistance score can be surmised.

Your body typically "saves" energy that you do not need by storing it as fat, with the intent of using it later. With high sugar consumption, there is a constant supply of energy, thus, there never is a "later." Fat remains and grows as more sugar is stored for "later." Triglycerides move around your vascular system and can damage the artery walls, potentially causing a hardening of the arteries (atherosclerosis) which increases the risk of strokes, heart attacks, and cardiovascular diseases.

HDL circulates through the bloodstream and carries small lipoproteins that act synergistically to cleanse the bloodstream. HDL performs the following beneficial functions:

- HDL cleanses and "takes up" the harmful LDL by circulating small assistant lipoproteins through the system.
- HDL recycles "bad" cholesterol by sending it to the liver, to be handled and reformed.
- HDL acts as a maintenance resource which repairs the internal lining of the blood vessels that have been damaged through a procedure known as "atherosclerosis" (hardening of the arteries).

Individuals who consume inordinate amounts of high-sugar foods and drinks, smoke, are inactive, or are obese, are more prone to developing heart disorders. Overall, people with low levels of HDL are more susceptible to developing heart disorders and other health issues, while those with high levels of HDL are much less likely to develop heart problems.

Sugar and the Immune System

In the 1970s, through his trials, scientist Linus Pauling demonstrated that blood cells require adequate amounts of Vitamin C. He discovered that when someone has a cold, high amounts of Vitamin C can treat it and heal it faster. Since both Vitamin C and sugar have similar chemical forms, they antagonize each other when blood sugar levels become elevated in the bloodstream. The two, factually, "rival" each other in penetrating the cell. Therefore, when higher amounts of sugar are present in the bloodstream, this prevents adequate amounts of Vitamin C from penetrating the cell.

Check your Vitamin C supplements. Some brands contain sugars, especially chewable Vitamin C. The sugar in the supplements is going to compete with the vitamin that you are taking for better health.

A heightened sugar level in the bloodstream can be very dangerous and, if left untreated, can cause nerve, tissue, or organ damage over time. Usually, when the body ingests food, these nutrients are broken down into glucose. The hormone insulin is then released into the bloodstream to manage blood sugar levels by transferring glucose into cells for energy. Over time, an elevated amount of sugar in the blood can lead to insulin resistance, where your cells do not respond properly to insulin, meaning that blood sugar levels cannot be controlled.

Common sugars have been demonstrated to worsen health problems, such as:

- Diabetes,
- Cancer,
- Cardiovascular problems,
- Arthritis,
- Osteoporosis,
- Infections,
- Development of gallstones.

In 1973, researchers published their work on how high amounts of sugar intake alter the function of immune cells, phagocytes.(Sanchez *et al.*) An important job of phagocytes is to engulf pathogens and protect the body from infections, however sugar intake decreases phagocytic activity. In the study, the number of phagocytes remained the same, it was the function that was affected by too much sugar.

Sugar and Cancer

Cancer cells live in low-oxygen, very acidic environments, and use sugar at a much more elevated pace than healthy cells do. Without becoming too technical, one of the issues with cancer cells is that they release lactic acid, thereby creating an acidic environment, in which cancer cells thrive.

> *After cancer treatments, I got peripheral neuropathy. I had no idea how much sugar I was consuming. It's everywhere! Dr Steph helped me get rid of all the excess sugar in my diet. Sugar may have given me cancer, but it won't ruin my life with neuropathy!*
>
> *~ Andy W*

As previously mentioned, the stored excess sugar becomes fat and obesity, according to the American Institute for Cancer Research, has been shown to be an increased risk factor for specific cancers.

- Breast (post-menopausal)
- Colorectal
- Endometrial
- Esophageal
- Gall Bladder
- Kidney
- Liver
- Mouth/Pharynx/Larynx
- Ovarian
- Pancreatic
- Prostate (advanced)
- Stomach

Cancer treatment protocols now aim to control blood sugar levels in multiple ways, in addition to promoting an alkaline environment. Physicians often recommend a healthy, low-sugar diet and exercise for patients with cancer, to the degree that this is possible.

Sugar and Mental Health

Sugar affects our mental health. Numerous trials examining the connection between sugar and the worsening of mental health disorders have been conducted by Malcolm Peet, an established and renowned researcher of mental health. Dr. Peet worked with patients suffering from schizophrenia.(Peet) Based on the outcomes of his studies, there is a clear association between elevated glucose levels and an increased risk of developing mental health problems, such as depression and schizophrenia.

Through comprehensive studies, Dr Peet determined that long-term inflammation can be triggered by a high intake of sugar, which suppresses the normal activity of the immune system. An abundance of sugar weakens the immune system. Additionally, evidence validates a connection between high sugar consumption and the aggravation of mental health disorders.

Sugar downgrades mental activity by hindering the function of an important growth hormone called brain-derived neurotrophic factor (BDNF). This leads to various chemical responses in the system that ultimately trigger long-term inflammation, which hinders the activity of the immune system and can lead to mental health or brain-related issues. When levels of the BDNF fall to lower ranges, there is an increased risk of developing depression or schizophrenia.

Several studies featured in the *British Journal of Psychiatry* demonstrate a connection between diets high in sugar and mental health issues, such as stress, anxiety, depression, and others. These trials demonstrated that people who regularly ingest high amounts of sugar are more likely to develop anxiety, depression, and possibly other mental health disorders. Additionally, sugar leads to a spike in adrenaline levels, again triggering episodes of induced stress, anxiety, and hyperactivity, with struggles to maintain focus.

Scientists have revealed that following a regular diet that is nutrient-dense and low in sugar balances mood levels, improves the ability to concentrate, and allows a person to deal with stressful situations more efficiently.

Addictive Attributes of Sugar and the Brain

Some individuals experience extreme cravings, and an urge for sweets or foods high in sugar and carbohydrates. Additionally specific changes in the brain have been observed when exposed to sugary foods. Animal trials have demonstrated alterations in the test animals' dopamine levels after eating sugar, such as seen in rats. Like drug addiction, rats provided with intermittent sugar offerings showed a remarkable increase in dopamine levels.

While people who frequently eat sugar do not experience the tremors, chills, or other harsh withdrawal symptoms that drug addicts experience, some people do experience intense cravings. Sugar cravings certainly exist, which can lead to excessive consumption of sugar, contributing to the development of excess body fat, obesity, heart issues and even death (in extreme cases).

Sugar cravings come from the brain's reward system, rather than the body's need for energy. As such, be prepared to face sugar cravings head on. Here are a few tips for over-coming sugar cravings:

- Drink lots of water. You may be feeling "hungry," instead your body is dehydrated.
- Avoid artificial sweeteners. These will cause you to consume more sugar.
- Eat more protein. When a craving hits, eat a hard-boiled egg instead of a sugary snack.
- Call a buddy. Engage in a good conversation and you will be distracted away from sugar.
- Eat regular, healthy foods. It is easy to fall into the starve yourself trap when you are trying to lose weight, however, this is not

the way to go if your goal is to have steady healthy weight.

- Go for a walk. If the cravings are too great, go for a brisk walk in the fresh air, clear your mind, overcome the craving.
- Stalk your kitchen with healthy snack foods. Have a stash of celery, cucumbers and carrots cut into bite-size pieces. These can satisfy the urge to snack with the satisfaction of a crunch.

Understanding that sugar cravings are just a need for rewards, you can find other ways to reward yourself. Remember your goals. Write them down or put them in your phone. Have a daily reminder of your goals and congratulate yourself for making it through each hour, day, week. By removing excess sugar from your diet, you are decreasing the inflammation cascade and improving your health.

The Inflammation Epidemic

Inflammation is the result of the immune system working to prevent infection by bacteria, or repairing damage caused by environmental factors, such as surgery. When an injury occurs, the body responds with four features of inflammation: pain, heat, redness, swelling.

Inflammatory disorders have reached epidemic proportions. These chronic conditions can greatly diminish your quality of life, such as respiratory issues, memory loss, allergic reactions, autoimmune disorders, skin problems, and many more. All these issues significantly affect Western populations.

In the past two decades, the frequency of degenerative diseases has been rising steadily. Inflammatory disorders have been affecting Americans at an alarming rate due to poor diet, inadequate sleep, and uncontrolled emotional or physical stress. The level of inflammation is at its peak and has almost become an epidemic.

What Are the Effects of Inflammation?

When a lesion gets inflamed, we can see the result with our eyes. However, inflammation is not always visible. The physical signs of "hidden" inflammation often emerge later - sometimes when it is too late.

Chronic, or long-term, inflammation can lead to multiple disorders, such as:

- Rheumatoid Arthritis,
- Polymyalgia Rheumatica,
- Bursitis,

- Tendonitis,
- Gouty Arthritis,
- DNA alteration that may lead to Cancer.

Additionally, osteoarthritis, fibromyalgia and some forms of neck and back muscle pain are suspected of being connected to chronic inflammation. A person who experiences long-term, uncontrolled inflammation is at higher risk for developing an inflammatory disorder and even accelerated aging.

Insulin resistance can also lead to inflammation. This is a result of consuming too many refined carbohydrates (refined sugars and starchy products like sweets, pasta, and white bread). People who are insulin-resistant are more inclined to being overweight and carrying excess fat around the abdomen, thighs, and buttocks. Studies have demonstrated that overweight individuals tend to produce more inflammatory chemicals than those who are not overweight. Moreover, as reviewed by Tristan Asensi *et al.* it has been demonstrated that sugar, refined foods, and processed foods can elevate the chemicals causing inflammation.

Stress and Inflammation

Chronic emotional, mental, and physical stress affects inflammation to a very high degree. When the system is exposed to stress, levels of cortisol rise within the body. Cortisol is a steroid hormone which is produced in response to high levels of stress, whether it be due to actual stressful events or an unhealthy diet or lifestyle. With inflammation, the stress reaction that develops to relieve the body from such circumstances is very hard to "switched off" again. Chronic stress is therefore linked to a chronic inflammatory response.

Chronic stress raises blood pressure which can lead to hypertension. Chronic high blood pressure also puts the blood vessels under tremendous amounts of stress. Stroke and heart failures are more common in people suffering from chronic inflammation, due to the non-stop inflammatory response of the body.

Stress can really eat you up! Thus, it is vital to learn ways of dealing with high-stress levels, and thus, avoid chronic inflammation. Some valuable relaxation methods include:

- Mild exercise,
- Yoga,

- Consuming healthy and nutrient-dense foods,
- Learning ways to keep emotional tranquility,
- Breathing exercises.

The traditional treatment protocol in response to inflammation is often a prescription for anti-inflammatory medicine. The commonly administered drugs in these cases are those that provide relief from pain.

Not long ago, the American Geriatrics Society removed nearly all non-steroidal and anti-inflammatory drugs (NSAIDs) from their guide of suggested pain-relievers for people aged 75 and older who experience chronic pain. It was discovered that these medications were prescribed more than necessary and could lead to adverse side effects in the elderly. Researchers have found that commonly used pain relievers such as ibuprofen, naproxen, and aspirin are not beneficial for chronic pain. Due to the research conducted on older individuals, researchers are now seeking to examine the effects of excessive use of NSAIDs in the younger generation too.

Anti-inflammatory drugs are aimed at lessening pain and discomfort, minimize swelling, and control symptoms of inflammation. Besides ibuprofen and aspirin, other common drugs prescribed include corticosteroids (cortisone, prednisone), and numbing pain relievers.

Anti-inflammatory drugs may demonstrate severe side effects with prolonged use. For instance, utilizing cortisone for extended periods can lead to serious problems with bone strength and integrity. Many chronic users of NSAIDs also develop stomach ulcers and internal bleeding, due to the mucus-blocking attributes of these pharmaceuticals. As such, the gastric wall is further exposed to stomach acid in those who take NSAIDs for longer periods.

Personalized functional medicine methods approach the matter of inflammation from a different perspective. Instead of prescribing synthetic drugs to inhibit inflammatory reactions, they suggest using vitamins or nutrients, and promote making positive lifestyle changes. While it is true that some vitamins and nutrients have powerful antioxidant and anti-inflammatory properties, they may not completely eradicate the problem. When dealing with inflammation a proper examination must be performed to determine the exact *cause* of inflammation. It is not beneficial to only treat symptoms, instead it is important to pinpoint the exact reason behind inflammation.

NSAIDs and Their Impact on Inflammation

As stated in the previous section, NSAIDs are often prescribed to reduce inflammation. They work by controlling the effects of prostaglandins. Prostaglandins are hormone-like substances released by the cells, that affect many bodily functions, including inflammation and pain. The enzyme responsible for making prostaglandins goes by the name "COX," short for cyclooxygenase. It is further divided into two enzymes: COX-1 and COX-2. Both trigger the release of prostaglandins, resulting in inflammation. NSAIDs block the activity of such enzymes. This eventually leads to long-term control of inflammation. However, the prostaglandins that protect the stomach lining and enhance blood clotting are also decreased, resulting in stomach ulcers and internal bleeding.

NSAIDs, when taken excessively, can interfere with the activities of COX-1 and hinder the cyclooxygenase pathways. When an NSAID like aspirin enters the system, COX-1 becomes acetylated, and its arachidonic acid pathway is hindered. This process of acetylation is responsible for aspirin's anti-clotting and blood-thinning effects.

Aspirin helps prevent blood clotting and eventually inhibits strokes and heart failures in people with a heightened risk of experiencing them. However, low-dose aspirin usage has been associated with kidney failure, stomach ulcers, irritable bowels, lethargy, increased bleeding tendencies, seizures and, ironically, increased risk of cardiovascular events.

Blood Assessments for Inflammation

In those who suffer from long-term inflammation, a certain protein is secreted by the inflamed regions and travels through the bloodstream. One of the standard blood tests to detect inflammation is a CRP (C-reactive protein) test. Elevated CRP levels are considered a sign of inflammation.

Homocysteine is an acid produced physiologically by the body when we consume excessive amounts of meat. Homocysteine levels in the blood can also be determined through blood tests. When homocysteine levels are abnormally high, the person is at a heightened risk of developing heart problems, atherosclerosis, heart failure, stroke, and Alzheimer's disease.

When the inflammation is hidden, resort to blood testing for the answers. CRP and homocysteine levels can be used to identify inflammation in the body. Follow up testing may be used to assess the effectiveness of lifestyle changes or treatments.

What is the Key Culprit Regarding Inflammation?

Researchers and medical experts keep examining the leading causes of inflammation. With so many contributing factors and issues linked to our diets, it is no surprise that gut inflammation plays a vital role. We will explain the matter in more detail in a later section, however, at this point, we should be aware that there is a clear connection between the gut and inflammation.

Gut disorders such as irritable bowel syndrome (IBS), Crohn's disease, and Celiac disease lead to a "leaky gut." The term "leaky gut" refers to a broken intestinal barrier. When the intestinal barrier is damaged, dietary proteins, gut pathogens and food-related chemicals can infiltrate the body. These circulating antigens contribute to the inflammatory cascade. If the barrier is not repaired, the inflammation will continue and could result in an inflammatory disorder such as allergies, arthritis, chronic heart problems and other clinical conditions.

Personalized functional medicine considers the triggering causes of a disorder rather than simply providing a "remedy" for treating the symptoms. Gut diseases and syndromes may originate from food sensitivities, physical or emotional stress, gut dysbiosis and other immune factors. It is vital to examine all these triggers when addressing chronic health issues.

By addressing inflammation from a more practical perspective, unlike allopathic or single treatment options, we can determine the triggering cause of this modern epidemic and thus be able to avoid it!

The Trouble with Statins

According to the CDC, between 2003 and 2012, the percentage of people of the age of 40 using cholesterol-lowing medication increased from 20% to 28%. By 2012, 93% of adults using cholesterol-lowering medication used a statin. Adults aged 40-64 with health insurance are more likely to be using a statin. Across the pond in the United Kingdom, around 74.3 million people are on a statin therapy. With so many people taking statins, it sounds like it must be some kind of wonder drug.

Statins do have some good qualities and one must weigh the pros versus the cons prior to embarking on a statin regimen.

USE OF STATINS PROS	USE OF STATINS CONS
• Lipid lowering effect • Pleiotropic effects • Improvement of endothelial function • Anti-inflammatory • Immunomodulatory effects • Anti-thrombotic effect	• Increase risk of neuropathy • Increased risk of myopathy • Increased risk of diabetes • Increased risk of hemorrhagic stroke • Muscle weakness, aches, and cramps • Stiffness • Tenderness

It is difficult to approve of statins, when it has been demonstrated that a low-fat, vegan diet works as well as a statin, without the possible side effects.

What Are Statins?

Statins, or HMG-CoA reductase inhibitors, are cholesterol-lowering drugs that are prescribed to patients with a history of, or who are deemed to be at risk of, cardiovascular complications. Statins mainly function by affecting the cholesterol synthesis pathways in the human body. Moreover, they also affect other metabolic processes and enzymes in the mitochondria, which are responsible for producing energy needed by the skeletal muscles to function, as well as sending and receiving messages or neural impulses by the peripheral nervous system.

Why Are They Prescribed?

The primary reason for prescribing statins is to lower cholesterol. Cholesterol can accumulate in the body for many different reasons, be it because of diabetes, obesity, or due to potential cardiovascular complications, like coronary heart disease, heart attacks, and heart failure. People with diabetes are, therefore, prescribed statins because they are believed to be at a greater risk of atherosclerotic cardiovascular disease. Researchers reiterate that statins can create a substantial risk for new-onset diabetes (normally connected to people over 50, who suddenly develop diabetes), but there is no consensus on the exact molecular mechanism.

Laakso *et al.* found that statin users had a 46% higher chance of developing new-onset diabetes, with a stark 24% increase in insulin resistance and a 12% decrease in insulin secretion. The most widely accepted mechanism for inducing new-onset diabetes is the ability of statins to reduce insulin secretion and sensitivity to insulin. An extensive analysis of studies encompassing 1.9 million diabetic patients found a clear correlation between a decline in glycemic control and atorvastatin intake.(Angelidi *et al.*) It is important to note that because patients with familial hypercholesterolemia have a mutated low-density lipoprotein receptor, or LDLR gene, they are protected against developing type-2 diabetes. Therefore, it does not make logical sense to continue prescribing these drugs to diabetic patients, solely as a precautionary measure against future cardiac complications.

Anomalies in human health could therefore be due to one or more reasons which are often associated. Statins may fix *one* aspect of the problem and yet ignore the bigger picture. Contemporary medicine strongly advocates personalized treatment, which considers the patient's predisposition to ailments. Such as diabetes, any history of cardiovascular complications, obesity, metabolic syndrome, and psychological stressors. Only then a treatment is proposed by a multidisciplinary team of professionals from different scientific specialties.

Statins, the Mediterranean Diet and Mortality

Statins are known to protect against cardiovascular complications and reduce mortality by 12%, but they do so at the expense of other metabolic processes. On the other hand, the Mediterranean diet has been shown to improve mortality by 37%. It also protects against diabetes, cardiovascular complications, and cancer. This debunks the overstated benefits of statins, but also the idea that merely lowering cholesterol helps protect against coronary heart disease.

What Impact Do Statins Have on Peripheral Neuropathy?

Patients with type-2 diabetes are susceptible to developing peripheral neuropathy. Statin users are up to 14 times more likely to develop peripheral neuropathy. What is the likelihood of a person with type-2 diabetes, who is on a statin, developing neuropathy? Min *et al.* found that diabetics using statins had an increased incidence of new-onset neuropathy than diabetics not using statins.

The paradoxical behavior of statins in the human body has led to a serious debate regarding their long-term effects. Medical treatments need to consider the human body's fundamental needs without eliciting serious damage. Today, you must seriously consider the pros and cons of statins.

Thus far, the discussion and scientific evidence are against the long-term use of heavy-dosage statin drugs. However, the increasing trend in sedentary lifestyles has caused increased concern regarding high cholesterol levels. These elevated cholesterol levels imply that statins will remain in the market despite their adverse consequences.

What Is an Effective Alternative to Reducing Cholesterol Without the Use of Statin Medications?

There are several over-the-counter alternatives to statins. One of the more common ones is niacin, which has been empirically demonstrated to decrease the secretion of LDL by inhibiting its precursor. In addition, niacin can also inhibit the secretion of triglycerides and HDL cholesterol. However, a controversial study, headed by the HPS2-THRIVE Collaborative Group, in 2014 found that long-term administration of niacin could lead to an increased risk of strokes and hyperglycemia. Nevertheless, niacin is an FDA-approved drug with formulations ranging from immediate, extended, and sustained release.

Ezetimibe is a protein inhibitor that blocks cholesterol absorption from the gastrointestinal tract and has been shown to result in a 17% reduction in LDL levels in patients suffering from hyperlipidemia.

Fabric acid has been demonstrated to decrease LDL and increase HDL cholesterol; however, it is not without its side effects. Fibrates can cause dyspepsia and gallstones.

Bile acid, which sequesters bile acid into an insoluble form that is later ejected from the body, helps lower the level of bile acids in the liver. This, in turn, causes an increased conversion of LDL to bile acids, thereby also increasing HDL and triglyceride levels. While it can be used as an alternative, its efficacy is only 30% compared to statins.

A more promising candidate for a potential replacement for statins is the antibody to a serine protease PCSK9, which can then decrease LDL concentrations significantly. Two such antibodies, alirocumab and evolocumab, have been shown to reduce LDL concentrations significantly and have good safety profiles. Their comparative efficacy with statins has yet to be established, but they remain good candidates for statin-free therapies.

In some cases, these alternatives may also cause side effects similar to, or worse than, those of statins. Except for perhaps PCSK9, the usage of the rest of the alternatives in clinical settings as reliable replacements for statins remains to be determined.

CHAPTER 4

EAT YOUR WAY OUT OF PAIN

M uch of the pain and inflammation from which an individual suffers is conditioned biochemically. Is there a way to naturally influence the body's chemistry to reduce pain and inflammation? The answer is yes! Some foods increase inflammation, while others can reduce it. Understanding this will allow you to make lifestyle changes that can reduce or even eliminate the need for taking painkillers.

The fact is that your lifestyle and food can affect how much pain you feel. Research published in the *Journal of the American Medical Association* (Esposito *et al.*) shows that the Mediterranean diet can protect the lining of blood vessels and reduce inflammation. In the study, chemicals that typically produce inflammation were reduced with this diet.

Boegman and Dziedzic documented the anti-inflammatory properties of diet and supplementation on elite rowers. This was first tested in 1996 on a group of rowers from the Danish Rowing Association. The study found that a combination of antioxidants and essential fatty acids could effectively treat the type of inflammation commonly known as "tennis elbow," and "golfer's elbow."

Antioxidants neutralize free radicals, limiting their destructive effects. Therefore, athletes should ensure they receive sufficient levels of antioxidants to protect themselves from stress injuries. Additionally, essential fatty acids are important as they promote the production of type 1 and type 3 prostaglandins in the body, which can neutralize pain and inflammation. Another aspect of your diet that can reduce pain and inflammation is the types of fats and oils you consume.

According to a study by Dr Sperling of Brigham and Women's Hospital, fish oil can reduce inflammatory substances produced by white blood cells. Sperling found that three months of supplementation reduced morning stiffness and tender joints. If you have an inflammatory condition, such as rheumatoid arthritis, the type of fat in your diet can affect the immune system's inflammatory response.

Foods That Can Lead to Inflammation

For those affected by inflammation, diets rich in carbohydrates and low in protein intake can be very destructive. We have witnessed multiple times that such high-carbohydrate and low-protein diets lead to inflammation and inflammatory disorders. In contrast, the opposite diet (low in carbohydrates and high in protein) keeps inflammation under control and all the associated negative side effects. Every individual body is unique, and thus it is essential to spot all the signs and symptoms we may experience when eating certain foods. Processed sugars and foods with a high glycemic index raise insulin levels and trigger an immune system response. Inflammatory mediators (prostaglandins and cytokines) react to insulin interactions and blood sugar levels. Studies reveal that when certain stressors occur, insulin triggers an inflammatory reaction within the body.

Some of the worst foods that can trigger an inflammatory response in the body are:

- Sugar/Sweets. High sugar consumption has been associated with obesity, inflammation, and chronic inflammatory diseases, such as diabetes mellitus.

- Cooking oils. Cooking and baking oils to avoid are corn, canola, soybean and "vegetable."

- Trans fats are typically found in junk food and fast-food meals and are associated with inflammation, resistance to insulin, and other chronic disorders.

- Non-organic milk and dairy products can also result in inflammation, especially in women, due to the hormones and allergen ingredients they contain.

- Eating red or processed meat, such as corned beef, steaks, lunch meat or canned beef is associated with immune reactions that lead to chronic inflammation. There is also a clear connection between processed meat consumption and the risk of cancer, backed up by many scientific studies.

Other types of foods suspected of causing inflammation are grains, flour, alcohol, synthetic food preservatives, and grain-fed meats. All the above foods should be avoided if any signs of inflammation turn up.

Concealed Sugars

Studies conducted by the University of Vermont's Nutrition Department found that only a small minority of Americans comply with the standard guideline of ingesting no more than 150 daily calories from sugar sources, as published by the American Heart Association (AHA). Those who adhered to the following AHA guideline show a decreased risk of developing heart disorders, as opposed to those who exceed the indicated levels of sugar intake per day.

Sugar is well-hidden in so many foods that we have no other option but to read the list of ingredients on every food label, to evaluate the amounts of sugar, or its forms, found in our food. Some food labels can be misleading or ambiguous, which increases the need for us to be aware of hidden sugars.

There are two general guidelines when it comes to deciphering food labels for sugar content:

- Words ending in -ose, as in "sucralose," "fructose," "dextrose," *etc.*
- Pay close attention to names like "evaporated cane sugar," or "evaporated cane juice."

Additionally, on many food labels (especially those for canned fruits, vegetables, and savory foods, such as meats or condiments) the word "syrup" often appears in the ingredients list. Furthermore, high fructose corn syrup (or glucose-fructose, isoglucose, and glucose-fructose syrup) is a sugar form made from starch. These sugars found in everyday foods are artificial and highly processed sugars that may lead to various health problems.

Processed sugars are the second leading cause of elevated sugars in our diets. However, the main source of hidden sugar in one's diet is not sweets, but soft drinks. These include colas, soda pops, juices, artificial fruit waters, and other drinks with high sugar content.

Following a diet refraining from excessive amounts of sugar can help stabilize our mood, stabilize blood sugar levels, and prevent various inflammatory conditions, thereby safeguarding our mental and physical health. The high amounts of concentrated, processed sugar found in our diets these days can be linked to a variety of health conditions. A naturally sweet, healthy diet is a much healthier and happier way to live!

An Anti-Inflammatory Diet

Much of the pain and inflammation from which an individual suffers is biochemically conditioned. Traditional pain medication provides relief by affecting biochemistry, so it is logical that other ways of influencing the body's biochemistry (such as diet and nutritional supplements) can affect pain and inflammation. By understanding which foods increase versus decrease inflammation, you may make positive lifestyle changes that reduce or even eliminate the need for painkillers.

Drink a Lot of Water Every Day

You need water to keep your cells hydrated and protected, eliminate waste, and ensure the health of your mucous membranes. The most important thing when it comes to drinking water is that water affects cartilage, which needs enough of it for your joints to function properly. Dehydration can cause excessive joint wear and may result in disc injury, so drink more water and fewer soft drinks, coffee, teas, or juices. Drink at least 8 glasses of water per day, or more specifically, calculate your ideal amount by weight. The rule of thumb is to drink, in ounces, 50% of your body weight in pounds. For example, if you weigh 200 pounds, ideally, you should be drinking 100 ounces of water per day. If you are exercising, you will need to drink additional water to replace what you lost during your workout.

Eat a Lot of Vegetables

You should eat at least fifty percent of your food intake in the form of vegetables. Vegetables can be high in fiber, vitamin C, folic acid, antioxidants, and minerals. Some practitioners believe that we do not live on the food we eat; rather, we live on the energy within the food we eat.

Vegetables are rich in antioxidants. You may have heard of bioflavonoids or carotenes; these are pigments that give fruits and vegetables their color, and they are antioxidants that protect your cells. Fiber in vegetables also reduces the absorption of fats and toxins. Eating enough fiber may help you lose weight and normalize your cholesterol and blood pressure. They nourish the normal gut flora, nourish the lining of the gastrointestinal tract, help produce vitamins, and inhibit yeast and other unwanted organisms from growing too abundantly. Vegetables also accelerate intestinal transit time, reduce gut toxicity, and prevent irritation of the gastrointestinal lining.

Vegetables contain minerals which can help prevent osteoporosis. They also contain folic acid, which is necessary to produce serotonin and thus prevent depression, increase energy, and reduce the risk of a heart attack. Minerals are essential enzymatic cofactors and are necessary for most of the body's vital functions.

Choosing organic and good quality vegetables is essential for eating more nutrients. With modern farming methods, many vegetables raised with insecticides or pesticides have lost minerals and thus, eating these foods can leave you hungry since you did not supply the proper amount of nutrients your body craves. Eating organic vegetables can reduce the risk of cancer and heart disease, increase energy and mental clarity, lessen the problems caused by intestinal and liver toxicity, and alleviate the symptoms of allergies, asthma, arthritis, skin issues, digestive ailments, chronic sinusitis pain, and other health conditions.

About Oils

Avoid fried foods, trans fats, partially hydrogenated oils, and hydrogenated oils. Hydrogenation is the process by which the food industry transforms liquid oils into solid fats (called "trans fats"). Although hydrogenated oils are responsible for various health issues, the food industry utilizes them as they give packaged foods a longer shelf-life than natural oils. Trans fats that have been linked to a range of health issues including an increase in pain and inflammation.

These oils chemically prevent the formation of natural anti-inflammatory substances that the body produces. In addition, muscle fatigue and skin problems have also been associated with effects stemming from hydrogenated oils.

Inflammation is the primary cause of most chronic diseases, and trans fats have been linked to a wide range of health issues due to their inflammatory capabilities. Women with higher levels of trans fatty acids in their cells are more likely to develop breast cancer than those with lower concentrations, as well as having a significantly increased risk of coronary heart disease. Furthermore, these fat molecules enter our cells and make them less resistant to chemicals, bacteria and viruses which can lead to further immune system problems. It has been proposed that the absorption of trans fatty acids into the brain and nerves can disrupt their normal functioning, leading to issues such as attention deficit disorder and depression. The fatty makeup of these tissues makes them particularly susceptible to damage from trans fats.

While some fats can be detrimental to your health, not all of them should be considered bad! Hydrogenated oils are found in a plethora of processed foods and snacks such as chips, cookies, cereals, and bread; they are also quite common in margarine (which is far more harmful than butter), mayonnaise and bottled salad dressings. To ensure you make the right dietary choices when it comes to fat, pay close attention to food labels. Permissible fats are raw (not roasted) nuts, extra virgin olive oil, fat from avocados and fish oil.

Avoid Refined Sugar

The average American consumes a staggering 60 pounds of sugar and an additional 40 pounds of other sweeteners every year. Refined sugar has been linked to various health issues due to its ability to increase insulin and adrenal hormone production. Excessive consumption causes inflammation since it increases insulin levels, leading to the presence of inflammatory chemicals. Furthermore, this type of sugar causes essential minerals to be depleted through the increased production of adrenal hormones.

Consuming too much sugar has dire consequences, as it depletes essential vitamins, such as Vitamin B and C, while simultaneously nourishing yeast and other single-celled organisms in your gastrointestinal tract. When these bad bacteria multiply, they produce toxins that irritate your gut lining further, as well as eliminate beneficial bacteria that offer great health benefits to you.

In addition to all of this, sugar also aggravates many emotional stressors!

Eating sugar causes an abrupt rise in blood glucose levels, resulting in the body producing more insulin. A consequence of this is extra insulin secretion, and an even greater craving for sugary foods. The excessive consumption of sugar in time leads to insulin insensitivity, prompting the pancreas to produce more and ultimately leading to insulin resistance, or type 2 diabetes. The higher one's daily intake of sugary foods, the closer one comes to endangering health!

A correlation has also been established between sugar consumption and hypercholesterolemia. Those suffering from Syndrome X (high cholesterol, high LDL, low HDL, and elevated triglycerides) commonly eat too much sugar with refined carbohydrates. Excessive consumption of sugar can have a detrimental impact on your overall health, from aggravating allergies and sinusitis, to leading to depression, asthma attacks and even cardiovascular disease.

Furthermore, it is also known for causing migraines, fatigue, and irritable bowel syndrome.

Avoid Refined Carbohydrates

The typical American consumes nearly half of their calories from refined carbohydrates. These are grains that have been stripped of essential nutrients such as fiber, vitamins E and B, minerals, and beneficial bacteria; the only thing left is their carb-load value. Unfortunately, many of these starches create health problems similar to those caused by sugar. As a result, it is important to be mindful when consuming any form of refined carbs since they can all present potential risks to your well-being. Not only do these carbs take up space in your stomach, making you feel full (but getting no nutrients), but they can also inhibit the performance of your digestive and endocrine systems over time. People often eat refined carbohydrates due to the misunderstanding that, because they are low in fat, or they are "complex carbohydrates" and therefore good for you.

Avoid Chemical Additives

Processed and pre-made foods often contain a wide array of additives to enhance flavor or prolong shelf-life. Unfortunately, the average American consumes an astounding 10 pounds of food-related chemical a year. Food chemicals, such as preservatives and food-colorings can have devastating effects on one's health. To ensure your well-being and longevity, avoid any food items you can which contain hazardous chemical additives; you will be happier (and healthier) as a result!

Eat Slowly and Chew Your Food Thoroughly

To ensure optimal digestion, chew your food properly instead of swallowing it whole. It is easier for the body to break down well-chewed food, and it ensures the enzymes from your saliva, that help with digestion, have a chance to work. If you give yourself enough time to properly chew each bite, that will greatly aid your digestive system. Otherwise, chewing your food poorly can lead to nutrient malabsorption and other related problems within the intestinal tract, not to mention the promotion of harmful bacteria growth within the intestines.

> *Dr Steph's Plate Rule is a game changer. I have my whole family following it and we are so much healthier now.*
>
> ~ Esperanza B

What to Eat and What Not to Eat

We have covered a lot of foods in this chapter. To sum it up, here is a handy chart listing what foods decrease inflammation and inflammatory foods you should avoid.

What to Consume	What to Avoid
Decreases Inflammation	**Increases Inflammation**
• Antioxidants	• Refined sugar, carbohydrates
• Essential fatty acids	• Vegetable, hydrogenated oils
• Fish oil	• Trans fats and fried foods
• Purified water	• Milk products
• Vegetables (preferably raw)	• Red and processed meats
• Willow bark	• Grains
• Curcumin	• Alcohol
	• Synthetic preservatives, food coloring and other chemical additives

When consuming an anti-inflammatory diet, remember to limit your salt intake and eat slowly, chewing the food well. Ideally, you chew enough so that what you swallow is very "watery." Practice conscious eating at every meal and snack.

Consuming raw foods is often more beneficial than cooked meals. Alcohol and caffeine consumption should be kept at a minimum. Rather than restricting the amount of food you consume, begin to evaluate your diet in terms of what will help sustain and fuel your body.

To get you started on your anti-inflammatory diet, here is a sample meal plan:

DAY 1	BREAKFAST	Apple with almond butter.
	LUNCH	Tuna (mix it with olive oil, chopped onion and celery). Serve it on celery stalks, carrot sticks, and cucumber slices. You can also include tomato and onion slices.
	DINNER	Sweet potato (you can use a small amount of clarified butter/ghee – or slice it and cook it in a casserole with sliced apples in pineapple juice), large green salad with oil and vinegar dressing, and mixed cooked vegetables.
	SNACKS	Any fruit, nuts or any vegetable.
DAY 2	BREAKFAST	Oatmeal.
	LUNCH	Turkey, large green salad.
	DINNER	Brown rice, cooked vegetables, large green salad.
	SNACKS	Any fruit, nuts or any vegetable.

DAY 3	BREAKFAST	Quinoa.
	LUNCH	Chicken vegetable soup, large green salad.
	DINNER	Chicken, large green salad, cooked vegetables.
	SNACKS	Any fruit, nuts or any vegetable.
DAY 4	BREAKFAST	Melon
	LUNCH	Hummus, tabouli, goat feta cheese [if dairy tolerant] and cucumber slices.
	DINNER	Beef vegetable soup, large green salad.
	SNACKS	Any fruit, nuts or any vegetable.
DAY 5	BREAKFAST	Vegetable omelet (chopped onion, spinach, tomatoes and bell peppers [if nightshades are not a problem for you]).
	LUNCH	Stir-fried vegetables and brown rice.
	DINNER	Broiled salmon, avocado and green salad.
	SNACKS	Any fruit, nuts or any vegetable.

Before embarking on a supplement regimen (antioxidants, omega-3s, willow bark, curcumin) it is best to consult a healthcare practitioner who is knowledgeable about anti-inflammatory supplements. The need for supplementation varies from person to person. Additionally, the quality of the product matters. You do not want to waste money on a supplement brand that is laden with chemicals, sugar, fillers, and poor quality of nutrients.

CHAPTER 5

THE BENEFITS OF OXYGEN AND EXERCISE

O xygen is the single most vital restorative element. Oxygen is a potent detoxifying agent, and an inexhaustible antibiotic resource that serves as the conductor of our immune system's orchestra. We require oxygen to stay alive. Without oxygen, our lungs cannot breathe properly, our heart cannot beat correctly, our brain is unable to think clearly, and our muscles become immobile.

Oxygen is unquestionably the most critical nourishment for our bodies. This essential substance powers every chemical process vital to human health and sustains our cells, providing energy to metabolize carbohydrates and regulating the body's pH levels. Oxygen also eliminates harmful toxins from the body, encourages breathing, improves immunity

101

against infectious organisms, and is an all-inclusive source of nutrition!

Some myths about oxygen are:

- <u>Myth #1</u> – Exercise increases oxygen intake and the body's oxygen content. It is just the opposite – the more strenuous the exercise, the more oxygen is consumed than is inhaled.
- <u>Myth #2</u> – Oxygen is only needed for the elderly or injured. If the elderly steadily utilized oxygen as a preventative approach in their younger years, they might not have to be on "medical grade oxygen" during their later years.
- <u>Myth #3</u> – Breathing higher levels of oxygen can and will hurt you. This is not true unless you have an extremely low pH level, where your body is acidic.
- Myth #4 – Running at high altitudes is the best way to get "fresh air." This is not the case. The higher the altitude - the lower the oxygen purity. A major oxygen killer is a strenuous activity at high altitudes.

Oxygen is not only the source of all life within our body, but also the source of our energy. Well, technically, adenosine triphosphate (ATP) is the source of energy production within our bodies.

The next section tells you everything you need to know about ATP.

What is ATP?

Adenosine triphosphate or ATP for short, could be called the "sugar lump" of a cell. It is the way your cell temporarily stores energy which can be released quickly, when needed. Without plenty of oxygen, ATP levels are not adequate. Consequently, our bodies do not function as well as they should. A steady stream of oxygen through our body helps the normal process of cellular development and breakdown, which provides a standard stream of energy through ATP, to get us through the day.

The problem is that most of us do not get the adequate supply of oxygen we need, for several reasons. Firstly, we seldom breathe correctly. Secondly, our posture often is not very conducive to proper breathing. Breathing, indeed, is one of the innate intelligence activities that our bodies do without us being consciously aware that it is happening.

However, we can appropriately control our ability to breathe deeply using the diaphragm.

Take a moment now and monitor your breathing. Are you taking slow, deep breaths that you can feel at the bottom of your stomach? If you are like most people, your breathing probably reaches the bottom of your chest and no further. Now, take a deep breath (keep your shoulders still, but expand your stomach). Take another. Are you starting to feel more energized? You should – this is what it feels like when your body receives sufficient oxygen.

Breathing properly is not that hard to learn, so how come most of us do not? Well, stress is one reason for poor breathing. Have you ever noticed that your breathing becomes shallower and faster when you are stressed or upset about something? This is fine if you are in a fight-or-flight situation where shallower breathing is necessary for fast running.

However, our society often places us in perpetual states of stress, meaning that all the wrong hormones are consistently dumped into our blood, causing us to go into a fight-or-flight mode. This means that our breathing becomes shallower, rather than diaphragmatic. This impacts our bodies very negatively.

Also, poor posture does nothing to help us breathe correctly. Instead of sitting or walking tall, with our shoulders back so our lungs can expand, we tend to slump over our computers, steering wheels, and phones. Yes, a lousy posture means bad curvature of the spine, but it also means that the lungs get scrunched up and cannot function optimally. This means that less oxygen is delivered to your body.

So, what is the problem with shallow breathing? Well, less oxygen in our blood results in an anaerobic, rather than aerobic, environment. In this environment, our cells must adjust to a lack of oxygen to survive; in short, they sub-mutate into lower-functioning cells. When cells are forced into an anaerobic environment it creates an ideal environment for various ills, including the possible proliferation of cancer. Not only that, but most bacteria, viruses, fungi, parasites, and other pathogens that contribute to diseases are anaerobic, and cannot live in environments with high oxygen levels.

Chronic exhaustion, fatigue and poor immune system function are just some side effects of lacking enough oxygen. Here is a list of problems we can expect when our bodies do not receive enough oxygen:

- Circulatory problems,
- Memory loss,

- Irrational behavior,
- Irritability,
- Poor digestion,
- Muscle aches and pains,
- Respiratory issues,
- Dizziness,
- Acidic stomach,
- Sadness/depression,
- Weakness,
- Fatigue.

Furthermore, the lack of appropriate oxygen levels in our body can contribute to the onset of cancer, heart disease, and stroke.

So, if we safely and correctly flood our bodies with oxygen, what happens to the offending toxins and microbes? They are eliminated!

Simple Deep Breathing Exercise

No equipment is necessary for this simple deep breathing exercise. Take the time to do this throughout the day for optimal effects. Lie down. Close your eyes. Place your hands on your torso, with the fingers spread and the fingers of one hand placed between the fingers of the other hand. Your hands should cover your lowest ribs. Breathe deeply through your nose filling your lungs, pushing out your stomach. The fingertips of each hand should now be lined up. This shows that your torso has expanded 2 or 5 inches depending on your body type! When you think you cannot get more air in, pull in a little more. Hold for 5 seconds. Slowly release the air through your mouth. When you think you have it all out, push out a little more. Hold for 5 seconds. Repeat. You can work up to holding in for 8 seconds and holding out for 7 seconds. Do this at least three times in sets of ten repetitions each day. They hardly take more than five minutes but reap enormous rewards!

> *My shallow breathing was a huge problem for me. After learning simple breathing exercises, at first, I found it hard to do them. I had to set alarms. However, once I realized the increased energy I got from them, I couldn't wait. Now I do them whenever I feel stressed or fatigued and my well-being improves immediately!*
>
> ~ Stella K

The longer you hold your breath, the more oxygen will fill your lungs and mix with your blood. What is even better is that this increases the levels of carbon dioxide in the blood vessels, which can lead to them widening and growing stronger. This is how people who exercise often have significantly higher levels of oxygenation when they are not active.

With blood vessels absorbing the maximum amount of oxygen, whether cycling, running, or simply relaxing with a book - these short yet powerful deep breathing exercises will give you immense energy and benefits.

Advanced Oxygen Intake

There are a few ways to rapidly increase the oxygen in your bloodstream. In our office we have a couple of tools to use. Both hyperbaric oxygen chambers and intravenous ozone therapy are great ways to give you an influx of vital oxygen.

Hyperbaric Oxygen Chamber

Recent interest in hyperbaric oxygen chambers as an adjunct therapy for neuropathy pain has inspired research with interesting results.

Hyperbaric oxygen chambers allow a patient to breath 100% oxygen under increased atmospheric pressure. Hyperbaric oxygen therapy (HBOT) has been shown to suppress pain precursors and thereby attenuate chronic nerve pain in rat models of chronic neuropathy with pain. (Zhao *et al.*, Liu *et al.*) Good news for rats!

Human studies have also been performed. One study's results indicated that the use of HBOT improved pain scores, pain-related symptoms, and quality of life.(Schiavo *et al.*) Well, that is good news for humans too.

Hyperbaric oxygen chambers can be expensive to buy. However, there are clinics and doctor's offices that have them for patients to "rent" by the half hour or hour. Always use a hyperbaric oxygen chamber under supervision.

Intravenous Ozone Therapy

Ozone, also called O3, consists of three oxygen molecules instead of two. When ozone hits the bloodstream, it separates into two components, peroxide, and oxygen. Think of ozone as cleaning and refreshing the body all at once.

Intravenous (IV) ozone oxidizes the bloodstream, thereby destroying foreign bodies, such as viruses. Many pathogens prefer an anaerobic (without oxygen), instead of an aerobic (with oxygen), bloodstream in order to thrive. So, you can understand how increasing the oxygen in your blood can rid you of any unwanted hitchhikers.

Recently Clavo *et al.* administered ozone to subjects with chronic pain, secondary to chemotherapy-induced peripheral neuropathy. Amazingly 6 out of 7 individuals realized improvement in chronic pain. The effects of IV ozone are usually felt immediately, but the healing capabilities of ozone therapy last from days to weeks. During this period, nerves receive oxygen and become revitalized. This is the start of nerve repair. In 2022, Zarief *et al.* conducted an ozone therapy study of patients with diabetic neuropathy. We anxiously await the publication of their findings, however, in our practice, we have seen our own clinical results.

Ozone can be administered in various ways. One common therapy is called Prolozone, in which ozone is injected into an affected area to reduce inflammation and energize the local blood vessels and capillaries. This therapy reduces pain and promotes the regeneration of tissues in the injected area.

The preferred delivery method of ozone for diabetics is IV. By using IV ozone, we get a greater distribution of ozone throughout the body, including the peripheral areas. The major side effect of IV ozone therapy is the immediate boost of energy a patient feels. The reason for this sensation is that the inefficient use and ineffective use of oxygen by the body is decreased due to restriction of circulation in the patient suffering from neuropathy. This ignites free radical damage, production of lactic acid and chronic degeneration of tissues. Vital nutrients, that are needed to repair damage cannot reach effected areas. Once we provide that oxygen source, the body comes alive, and the patient feels that energy.

> Ozone Therapy has been phenomenal! I had my first treatment in 2018, skeptical of the outcome, I tried it anyway. I researched the benefits of the therapy and thought it couldn't hurt and Oh Boy was I right. Prior to my initial treatment my Eye Doctor told me I would need reading glasses, but immediately following only my first treatment, I no longer needed them. I also have psoriasis in my scalp and immediately following my second treatment, the psoriasis cleared up. I also notice I have more energy, healthier skin and no more tingling in my arms and fingers. Ozone along with the support of the staff here at Living Health, has completely changed my life. It's unfortunate that modern medicine doesn't offer this therapy because it works for EVERYTHING!
>
> ~ Ms Snowden

The Benefits of Breathing Right

After a routine session of deep breathing, you will feel energized all over. When utilizing abdominal breathing, you are forcing the diaphragm to enlarge your lungs for maximum capacity. There are many benefits when you work your lungs to their total capacity.

- Increased oxygenation in the blood helps remove toxins from your body's environment.
- Greater levels of absorption and assimilation of foods – and better digestion overall.
- An improved nervous system means better communication between the brain and your cells.
- Rejuvenation of the hormonal glands (especially the pineal and pituitary, which regulate brain function). Some people feel "smarter" after exercising, or after deep-breathing yoga. This is not their imagination – it is the brain getting more oxygen which, in turn, stimulates these two essential glands.
- A massaging effect on the heart and abdominal organs increases blood circulation and improves their effectiveness.

The excellent news about this is that it takes so little effort. Just a little concentration will net you all the above benefits!

Exercise and Neuropathy

Exercise has many benefits. This is not news. However, with modern, stressful lifestyles it can be difficult to find time for exercise, thus perpetuating an unhealthy being.

Routine exercise may enhance the recovery from, and/or reduce some of the symptoms associated with peripheral neuropathy. Aerobic exercises (brisk walking, swimming, bicycling) move large muscle groups, which require more oxygen, whin causes you to breathe deeply. Aerobic exercise causes a release of endorphins (our happy chemicals), which act as natural pain killers.

In a study on diabetic neuropathy, diabetics engaged in aerobic exercise training had developed significantly less sensory and motor nerve dysfunction.(Balducci *et al.*) Balance training can alleviate the feeling of tightness in muscles and joints. Regular balance training can improve balance thereby preventing falls.

For improving strength and stability Tai Chi is recommended. However, if Tai Chi sounds daunting, there are beginning stretching and balance exercises, provided by Healthline, that you can use to get started on less tightness and better balance. It is always recommended to stretch before exercising to prevent injury to muscles and tendons. Stretching warms up the muscles and tendons, increases circulation to the area, and prepares the body for exercise.

Calf stretch

- Place one leg behind you with your toe pointing forward.
- Take a step forward with the opposite foot and slightly bend the knee.
- Lean forward on the front leg while keeping the heel on your back leg planted on the floor.
- Hold this stretch for 15 seconds.
- Repeat three times per leg.

Seated hamstring stretch

- Sit on the edge of a chair.
- Extend one leg in front of you with your toe pointed upward.
- Bend the opposite knee with your foot flat on the floor.
- Position your chest over your straight leg and straighten your back until you feel a muscle stretch.
- Hold this position for 15 to 20 seconds.
- Repeat three times per leg.

Side leg raise

- Using a chair or counter, steady your balance with one hand.
- Stand straight with feet slightly apart.
- Slowly lift one leg to the side and hold for 5 to 10 seconds.
- Lower your leg at the same pace.
- Repeat with the other leg.

As your balance improves, try this exercise without holding onto the counter.

Calf raise

- Using a chair or counter, steady your balance.
- Lift the heels of both feet off the ground so you're standing on your toes.
- Slowly lower yourself down.
- Repeat for 10 – 15 reps.

Routinely engaging in stretching and balance training, you will see an improvement in your neuropathy symptoms.

Exercise with Oxygen Training (EWOT)

Our ability to transfer oxygen efficiently into our cells weakens over time, making us more susceptible to illnesses and diseases. When a person is only thirty, the amount of oxygen that reaches their cells is significantly higher than when they are seventy, about 55 millimeters for the former, and just 35 millimeters for the latter. As people grow older, however, there is a decrease in pressure regardless of the volume of oxygen present. This means that although it may seem like they are getting enough oxygen intake, eventually they become deficient due to insufficient pressure to make use of what's available.

Aging is not the only issue here. The increase in air pollution, namely carbon dioxide, decreases the amount of oxygen intake. Thus, if you live in an area of high air pollution, adequate oxygen intake may be a major health problem for you.

A remarkable solution has been uncovered, known as "EWOT" (Exercise With Oxygen Therapy). This innovative discovery helps boost arterial pressure back to its youthful levels. With EWOT, oxygen intake during exercise is increased, which results in greater circulation of the body and enhances blood flow, by forcing more oxygen into the capillaries. By utilizing this breakthrough method regularly, one can help their arteries return to their former youthful glory!

By boosting pressure back into the capillaries, EWOT repairs and restores their transferring abilities. Its remarkable effectiveness has been proven for a wide range of conditions due to its ability to greatly improve oxygen delivery, vital to tissue repair and improvement. After all, tissues must have oxygen to stay healthy!

EWOT is simple to use, affordable, and highly effective, allowing one to increase oxygen levels in their blood plasma with only 15 to 20 minutes of practice each day. This not only makes it convenient for everyone, but also offers long-lasting benefits that will keep one healthy throughout their life. With EWOT, you can get a full-body workout while breathing in oxygen-enriched air from your own Personal Portable Oxygen Bar.

You have the option to use a treadmill, stationary bicycle, an upper body ergometer/bicycle, or light weights to perform easy bicep curls, crunches, and cross-crawl exercises that are suitable for all users. For those of you who are in good physical health and have healthy joints, with no heart disease or other medical issues, a stationary bike could be the perfect way to begin your workout journey.

Remember, this is not about reaching top speed. Start out easily; at about two miles per hour (you can check your speed on the bike's speedometer). Additionally, for extra safety, wear a heart rate monitor. Most sporting goods stores have plenty of different heart rate monitors available. Follow your body's cues, and if you feel lightheaded or weak, stop immediately. Make sure to keep a good posture; no slouching when inhaling. Instead, sit up straight and look upward when inhaling.

Pay attention to your breathing. You will soon start noticing how wonderful it is when you deeply and slowly breathe in oxygen-enriched air. It is important not to let the simplicity of the process of EWOT fool you.

While exercising, these benefits can occur:

- The oxygen content of your blood increases,
- Your heart rate increases,
- More blood with higher oxygen content gets pumped throughout your body,
- More oxygen gets delivered faster to your brain, your heart, and various parts of your body.

EWOT helps deliver a necessary supply of oxygen to vital parts of our bodies; consequently, producing remarkable changes that can last a lifetime. Below are just some of the conditions or ailments from which users of EWOT have experienced relief:

- Chronic pain,
- Neuropathy,
- Balance issues,
- Dizziness,
- Weakness in joints,
- Fibromyalgia,
- Blood pressure problems,
- Vision problems,
- Immune function problems,
- Mood issues.

This breakthrough process can be effective in nearly every area of life, in terms of health and wellness.

CHAPTER 6

HOCATT WELLNESS SYSTEM

A perfect lifestyle naturally includes proper nutrition, regular exercise and detoxification, effective stress management, and healthy sleep. However, is not always easy to maintain as life tends to get in the way. Hence, a lifestyle compensator, such as HOCATT, can assist in achieving a healthier state within a short period of time.

The acronym HOCATT represents Hyperthermic Ozone and Carbonic Acid Transdermal Therapy. It refers to a technology that incorporates a variety of treatment modalities, to maintain the vitality of healthy individuals and improve the health of patients with chronic conditions. HOCATT was first designed by Andre Smith in 2002 and has since become an incredible therapeutic tool.

The component terms of the HOCATT system are briefly described below.

Hyperthermia

Hyperthermia is a state in which there is an increase in the body's internal temperature. This condition increases the body's metabolic processes and subsequently eliminates pathogens (infection-causing microorganisms) from the body.

Ozone

Ozone is a colorless therapeutic gas commonly referred to as 'super oxygen' because it comprises three atoms of oxygen, rather than the usual two. This therapeutic gas possesses a positive charge that allows for its oxidative effect (via neutralization) on several compounds with negative charges, such as organic compounds like toxins and foreign cells, and microorganisms.

Carbonic Acid

Carbonic acid is generated from carbon dioxide's interaction with steam. It gains entrance into the lymph system in the body through the pores. This compound stimulates the uptake and conveyance of oxygen into the cells, which causes the blood vessels to dilate, resulting in increased blood circulation. More importantly, carbonic acid shifts the body from a sympathetic (fight-or-flight) state to a parasympathetic (rest-and-digest) state. This treatment has been shown to help lower blood pressure.

Transdermal Therapy

Transdermal therapy refers to the mode of delivery of the therapeutic components of the HOCATT system. It refers to the passage of these components across skin membranes to general body circulation.

HOCATT is a breakthrough concerning health technologies that holistically improves health and vitality. It is a time, energy, and resource-saving non- invasive method of detoxification. It also aids in reinvigorating the body, through thermal, electrical, and mechanical energies. The HOCATT concept is distinct because it is an all-inclusive system incorporating several treatment modalities. It can stimulate multiple body systems at once to achieve an optimal state. Moreover, it is easy to use and produces noticeable results after the first or second session.

A typical HOCATT session lasts for about 25 to 30 minutes. The patient sits in the HOCATT machine with the head protruding from it, while the doors of the machine are closed. A neck cape is tied around the neck of the patient to prevent the escape of steam, ozone, and other gases. Pure, humidified oxygen is also supplied through an oxygen jet into the nose and mouth. Appropriate concentrations of a mixture of warm steam, carbonic acid, and ozone is then circulated throughout the sealed chamber. This mixture causes the blood capillaries to dilate, and the transdermal delivery of ozone is promoted by carbonic acid. The gradual rise in body temperature and the systemic increase in oxygen levels increase blood circulation and improve general well-being.

> *The HOCATT is great. I feel relaxed and less stressed when I get out of the HOCATT. Not to mention how much better I feel after the toxins have been released from my body. I sleep better, and my whole outlook has improved.*
>
> *~ AA*

Component Therapies of the HOCATT System

The therapies incorporated in the HOCATT system include:

1. Ozone therapy,

2. Carbonic acid therapy (CO_2 and steam),

3. Aromatherapy,

4. Light-emitting diode (LED) light and color therapy,

5. Passive exercise with oxygen therapy,

6. Far infrared therapy (FIR),

7. Whole-body hyperthermia,

8. Frequency-specific microcurrent therapy (FSM),

9. Pulsed electromagnetic field therapy (PEMF).

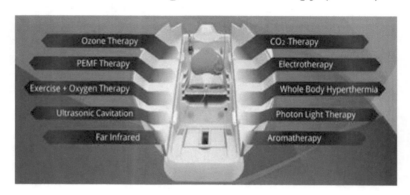

1. Ozone Therapy

Ozone is a gas ranging from colorless to blue. It is an energized form of oxygen and is one of medicine's most prominent therapeutic agents. Ozone therapy has been used singly for neuropathic pain. Once ozone enters the bloodstream, it depresses inflammatory chemicals, such as nuclear factor kappa-light-chain-enhancer of activated B cells (NF-κB) and increases anti-inflammatories such as transforming growth factor beta-1 (TGF-B1). TGF-B1 decreases the hypersensitivity associated with nerve damage.

As we are writing this book, Dr Zarief, at Assiut University, is writing and publishing the results of a 2022 clinical trial using ozone therapy in patients with diabetic neuropathy.

Ozone's general mechanism of action involves the formation of reactive oxygen species that act to enhance cellular and biological processes. Ozone eventually reverts to oxygen after use, making it an eco-friendly oxidant. Transdermal ozone is the therapeutic application of ozone into the skin, through the pores.

Benefits of Transdermal Ozone

The overall benefits of transdermal ozone in HOCATT therapy include the following:

- Inactivation of Microbes. Microorganisms such as bacteria, viruses, fungi, and parasites are inactivated by transdermal ozone, through a direct oxidative effect. The positive charge of ozone neutralizes the negatively charged microbial cells, leading to their destruction. Also, ozone facilitates the eradication of active infections, as microbes are incapable of producing antioxidant enzymes.

- Immune Support. Most individuals are constantly exposed to an infinite amount of chemicals and pathogens that threaten the immune system. The immune system is the body's defense against intruders. Thus, the successful invasion of the body by these substances has harmful effects. Many of these can trigger immune destruction of the peripheral nerves, therefore, balancing the immune system is vital for nerve protection and healing. Transdermal ozone helps circumvent this situation by boosting the immune system and ensuring the retention of its integrity to combat exposure to these foreign agents.

- Detoxification of the Body. Transdermal ozone binds toxins, chelates heavy metals, and scavenges free radicals. This action promotes their destruction and elimination from the body, and many of these toxins are damaging to the peripheral nerves.

- Improvement of General Well-Being. Ozone therapy increases the body's circulation and energy on a cellular level, by enhancing the production of the energy currency of cells - adenosine triphosphate (ATP) - by the mitochondria. It also promotes tissue utilization of oxygen. Nerves need ATP to function, and they also need oxygen and nutrients delivered to them daily to heal and repair.

- <u>Promotion of Hormones and Enzyme Production</u>. The production of endogenous proteins, such as hormones and enzymes, is stimulated and normalized during transdermal ozone therapy.

- <u>Adjunctive Therapy in Cancer Treatment</u>. Ozone therapy has been shown to modulate the immune system and reverse oxygen deficits in the body. These benefits have been shown to suppress the growth of tumor cells and improve immune function.

- <u>Anti-inflammatory Effects</u>. Ozone therapy reduces inflammation by oxidizing and inactivating inflammatory mediators, such as prostaglandins.

- <u>Stimulation of The Body's Natural Antioxidant System</u>. The efficiency of antioxidant enzymes that scavenge free radicals in the body is enhanced.

- <u>Analgesic Effects</u>. It relieves pain by calming and soothing the nerves.

- Promotion of Cognition. It also increases memory and mental functioning.
- Anti-aging Effects Transdermal ozone reduces stress and anxiety and helps keep the skin rejuvenated. The increase in antioxidant system efficiency by ozone also destroys free radicals, that are implicated in the aging process.

2. Carbonic Acid Therapy

Carbonic acid is formed by reacting carbon dioxide (CO_2) and water (steam). Carbonic acid is essential for the uptake and delivery of oxygen into cells for optimal function. It prevents hypoxic conditions, impaired protein repair, and improper cell growth that results from an inadequate supply of oxygen to the cells. This is essential for the repair and regeneration of peripheral nerve tissue.

In a HOCATT therapy session, CO_2 is supplied into the chamber from outside, while steam is generated within. The interaction of steam with CO_2 produces carbonic acid that is then absorbed through the skin.

Benefits of Carbonic Acid Therapy

- Increased supply of oxygen to cells.

- Increased blood circulation throughout the body.
- Considerably fast absorption of ozonated products into the body compared to a regular sauna.
- Decreased blood pressure due to the dilation of blood vessels and capillaries.
- Reduction in stress and anxiety due to its relaxing effects on the muscles, mind, and central nervous system.
- Anti-inflammatory effects help to calm nerves and soothe the pain due to their natural anti- inflammatory properties.
- Stimulation of the autonomic nervous system and calming the central nervous system allows for tissue regeneration and relaxation of the body.

3. Aromatherapy

Aromatherapy is the application of aromatic compounds (such as essential oil infusions) through the sense of smell to achieve therapeutic benefits. Necessary oil infusions are fragrant and volatile preparations of essential oils with steam. These oils are obtained from aromatic plants, by utilizing heat and pressure treatments.

Essential oils (EOs) consist of secondary metabolites and may be derived from aromatic plant parts such as leaves, fruits, flowers, bark, roots, *etc.* Examples of such plants are lavender, eucalyptus, bergamot, peppermint, and tea tree.

Although anecdotal evidence exists, clinical research data on the use of EOs for neuropathy is lacking. Dosage guidelines very dramatically in the literature. Even so, those who utilize Eos in diffusers, as inhalants, or topically, know how effective they can be.

EO infusions possess incredible healing abilities. Their high volatility predisposes them to rapid absorption and enhances their distribution into the bloodstream. If you are new to using EOs, it is best to work with a professional on how to use them safely and effectively.

Benefits of Aromatherapy

- Detoxification of the body.
- Management of stress, tension, and anxiety by calming down central and peripheral nerves.
- Improvement of cognition and mental clarity stimulation via altering specific brainwaves.

- Alleviation of insomnia and improvement in sleep quality because of its soothing effects on the entire body.
- Anti-inflammatory and analgesic effects.
- Antimicrobial activities against bacteria, fungi, viruses, and parasites.
- Antioxidant and age-slowing effects.
- Relief of respiratory distress with colds, bronchitis, coughing, asthma, etc.
- Eradication of skin problems, and promotion of wound healing.
- Improvement of quality of life.

4. Light-Emitting Diode (LED) Light and Color Therapy

LED light and color therapy are non-invasive procedures for treating many disease conditions. Red to near-infrared LEDs have been shown to promote nerve regeneration. Thus, the therapy can both ease pain and repair damage.

In this therapeutic technique a skin-friendly, visible light of different wavelengths is used, which does not cause harm to the cells or tissue.

LED light of different colors penetrates various skin strata to stimulate the body's natural repair mechanisms. The light colors include blue, yellow, red, green, indigo, orange, and violet. The HOCATT session exposes the patient to all these forms of LED light colors.

Benefits of LED Light and Color Therapy

- Violet aids in alleviating insomnia and minimizes stress and anxiety through its sedative effect on the central nervous system.
- Blue combats infection and inflammatory conditions. In addition, it causes easy destruction of bacteria and improves acne conditions by reducing oil production by the sebaceous gland.
- Red increases blood circulation and energy levels.
- Green relieves cardiovascular disorders, peptic ulcer disease, flus, headaches, and migraines.
- Yellow stimulates mental focus and aids in the relief of pain associated with indigestion and constipation.
- Orange is mainly effective in the respiratory system, in treating asthma and bronchitis.

5. Passive Exercise with Oxygen Therapy

Oxygen therapy involves breathing in pure, 100%, concentrated, and humidified oxygen and a passive form of exercise. The procedure boosts oxygen saturation, increases oxygen delivery to the body, and allows oxygen to deeply penetrate damaged tissue. These actions accelerate the body's natural healing process and promote maximal performance. Oxygen therapy with exercise is potent as it improves the quality of life of a patient, by keeping the muscles and entire body system active and revitalized.

Benefits of Oxygen Therapy with Exercise

- Improvement in blood flow and tissue repair.
- Adjunct to physiotherapy for treating acute injuries and chronic muscle pains.
- Alleviation of pain and inflammation during the session.
- Preservation of mitochondrial ability to generate energy. This action is significant because every cell in the body requires energy for effective functioning.
- Increase in energy levels for utmost performance of day-to-day activities.
- Promotion of oxygen absorption and lung function.

- Burns of up to 30% calories.

6. Far Infrared Therapy (FIR)

Far infrared therapy is an invisible component of the electromagnetic spectrum with a wavelength longer than visible light. FIR is a low-energy therapy form where light waves penetrate the human body, transform into heat energy to elevate the temperature, and gently activate major primary functions. Approximately half of the power generated by the human body is naturally infrared. FIR is considered entirely safe and although FIR is invisible, patients can feel it in the form of pure heat.

FIR therapy can heal damaged nerves by increasing blood circulation and triggering the release of nitric oxide (NO). NO promotes healing. Nerve function recovery is possible using FIR.

FIR waves heat the body directly without necessarily heating the surrounding air in a typical FIR therapy session. This operation renders it more beneficial when compared to conventional heat therapies, where the surrounding air is initially heated before it warms up the entire body. During HOCATT therapy, FIR therapy is radiated from the chamber into the feet and back, to easily circulate the infrared waves throughout the entire body.

Benefits of the FIR Therapy

- Increased oxygen supply to damaged tissues.
- Promotion of blood circulation in the arterial and peripheral vessels.
- Improvement of endothelial function through inhibiting tumor necrosis factor (TNF) and interleukin-6 (IL-6). Nitric oxide synthase production in the endothelium is thus promoted, and endothelial function subsequently improves.
- Reduction of oxidative stress, a process that accelerates the development of degenerative diseases and aging.
- Relief of pain and inflammation.
- Detoxification of the body by the neutralization of biological and environmental toxins.
- Improvement of symptoms for several diseases such as neuropathy, chronic fatigue syndrome, fibrocystic breast disease, fibromyalgia, *etc.*

7. Whole-Body Hyperthermia

Whole-body hyperthermia is a treatment modality that increases the core body temperature to about 40-45°C (104-113°F). The procedure aids in destroying harmful cells with no injury to normal tissues. It acts by activating specific mechanisms that diminish protein (hormones and enzymes) damage at the molecular level, thereby promoting the average growth of cells and tissues. It also cleans and detoxifies the entire body for optimal wellness.

Benefits of Whole-Body Hyperthermia

- Increase in efficiency of the natural antioxidant and repairing systems.
- Enhancement of mental clarity.
- Growth in the immune system's efficiency through producing white blood cells that fight against diseases.
- Enhanced blood flow and circulation increase the body's metabolic processes.
- Facilitation of a quick recovery after exercise by promoting the elimination of lactic acid, the culprit responsible for muscle fatigue.
- Adjunct to chemotherapy and radiotherapy in cancer treatment. Whole-body hyperthermia promotes the shrinkage of

tumors and apoptosis of malignant cells by heat stress.

- Fibromyalgia treatment. Fibromyalgia is a condition mainly characterized by musculo-skeletal pain with alterations to memory, mood, and sleep. In Germany, Walz *et al.* studied fibromyalgia patients who received whole-body hyperthermia. Walz concluded that participants experienced rapid pain relief and had an improved quality of life.

8. Frequency-Specific Microcurrent Therapy (FSM)

Frequency-specific microcurrent therapy is a form of electrotherapy. Electrotherapy itself refers to the application of electrical energy to achieve therapeutic benefits. The HOCATT supplies this energy through metal footplates.

Electrotherapy explores the fact that every cell in the body is electrically active, as a certain amount of electrical energy is required for the optimal functioning of any cell. However, human energy may become dissipated by poor nutrition, inadequate oxygen supply, exposure to toxic chemicals, and activities of free radicals. Hence, there is a need for an energy compensator such as electrotherapy procedures. Our peripheral neuropathy patients receive many forms of electrotherapy, including neuropathy frequency settings, in each HOCATT session.

Frequency-specific microcurrent therapy has mainly found application in treating neurological and musculoskeletal problems, offering tissue regeneration and pain relief benefits, respectively. The electrical energy generated during the procedure may stimulate or activate the body's physiological state, leading to cell membranes' depolarization and generating an action potential. Hence, pain relief is achieved by stimulating the sensory nerve fibers.

Benefits of Frequency-Specific Microcurrent Therapy

- Frequency-specific microcurrents cause the contraction of skeletal muscles, thereby serving as a form of passive exercise that recharges the body's cells with energy.
- It is a delicate procedure that provides both anti- inflammatory and analgesic effects.
- It accelerates tissue regeneration.
- It also activates the body's metabolic processes.

9. Pulsed Electromagnetic Field Therapy (PEMF)

Pulsed electromagnetic field therapy is a bio-magnetic technology that utilizes low-frequency, but high-intensity, electromagnetic energy to provide medical treatment. First, it provides the entire body with the flow of Earth's natural magnetic waves. These waves are subsequently transformed into electrical energy that charges the body's cells to an optimal state.

Pulsed electromagnetic field therapy is a procedure with incredible energy-generating abilities that reinvigorates the human body and allows for optimal performance of day-to-day activities.

Benefits of Pulsed Electromagnetic Field Therapy

- Increase cellular function and efficiency allowing for tissue regeneration and repair.
- Optimization of cellular energy levels and vitality.
- Increase in cellular metabolic processes.
- Promotion of blood flow and circulation.
- Enhanced delivery of oxygen and nutrients into the cells.

- Immune support through the stimulation of antibody production by the immune system.
- Improved removal of metabolic waste products from the cells.
- Prevention of the effects of damaging electromagnetic radiation from mobile phones, computers, microwave ovens, *etc.* These radiations damage cell membranes and render the body susceptible to illnesses.
- Prevention of muscle fatigue and rapid recovery after exercise.
- Immediate and long-lasting alleviation of pain
- Reduction of stress, tension, and anxiety.
- Stimulation of muscle contractions, which serves as passive exercise to promote the circulation of lymph fluids throughout the body.
- Complete detoxification of excretory organs such as the liver and kidneys.
- Promotion of general well-being and increase in quality of life.

Who Benefits from the HOCATT Wellness System?

The HOCATT wellness system is a beneficial therapy for everyone seeking to improve their quality of life. Healthy individuals that seek to promote and maintain their vitality can utilize it to ensure the maximal performance of their daily activities. It may also be a suitable adjunctive therapy for patients battling various health disorders, such as neuropathy, microbial infections, allergic disorders, diabetes, cancer, vascular disorders, degenerative diseases, *etc.*

Professional and amateur athletes alike can benefit from the HOCATT wellness system, as it can boost athletic performance by reducing muscle spasms and pain which culminates in muscle fatigue. Likewise, it increases stamina and intensifies endurance. Regular use of HOCATT can help athletes recover more quickly after long days of training.

In addition, the wellness system effectively reduces weight in overweight patients with a predisposition to obesity, as patients can burn up to 600 calories per session. In such patients this reasonably lowers the risk of obesity-facilitated disorders such as strokes, dyslipidemia, hypertension, type 2 diabetes, coronary heart disease, *etc.*

Expectations from HOCATT

The HOCATT therapy is a phenomenal and revolutionary therapy with the shot-gun effect, since it utilizes multiple technologies in one session that are perfectly sequenced to enhance and amplify the activities of one another. Not only does this therapy offer incredible therapeutic benefits, but it may also be a shortcut to optimal wellness.

Finally, the HOCATT wellness system is a suitable complementary therapy to conventional treatments and is expected to improve the patient's quality of life. The synergistic benefits of the system's components keep all the body systems active and running optimally. With HOCATT patients can effectively get reinvigorated with energy to go about their daily activities.

In addition, they can effectively achieve whole-body detoxification, manage stress, and experience better relaxation. Finally, patients can heal damaged nerves and eliminate nerve pain.

CHAPTER 7

RED-LIGHT THERAPY
FOR NEUROPATHY

T oday red and near-infrared light therapy has become popular healthcare intervention. Elite professional athletes, Hollywood celebrities, renowned skincare specialists, world-class fitness trainers, and natural health specialists, utilize red-light therapy in their treatment modalities or healthcare plans. It can also aid those suffering from neuropathy.

NASA utilized it in the 1980s to grow plants in space. They discovered that the strong light from red-light-emitting diodes (LEDs) aided plant cells in their development of and ability to photosynthesize. Because of this, the medical potential of red-light therapy (RLT) was studied further, with special attention given to its capability to enhance energy production within human cells. It was considered a possible effective treatment for delayed wound healing, muscular dystrophy, and bone density loss experienced by astronauts during space travel.

Here on Earth, the application of LEDs to the fluids produced from nerve stumps, after nerve injury, promoted mitochondrial oxidative metabolism. Those are some complex words. In simple terminology, the LEDs counteracted the damaging effects and allowed for nerve regeneration.

RLT, also known as photo-biomodulation (PBM), low-level light therapy (LLLT), cold laser therapy, soft laser therapy, photonic stimulation, or low-power laser therapy (LPLT), is referred to as a "photodynamic treatment" when combined with photosensitizing drugs. In this case, red light acts as an activator for the medicine.

This therapy exists in a variety of forms. In beauty salons, one can find red light beds that reduce cosmetic skin problems, such as stretch marks, blemishes, and wrinkles. In medical settings, RLT can help treat conditions like psoriasis, slow-healing wounds, and side effects of chemotherapy. Additionally, there are indications that RLT might be an effective treatment modality for complications associated with diabetes, such as peripheral neuropathy and diabetic wounds.

The Science Behind Red Light Therapy

Red-light therapy uses wavelengths that superficially penetrate human tissue, with the first 2 cm absorbing approximately 80% of the energy. The optimal wavelength range for best results is between 650 and 850 nm. This light can penetrate the epidermis (top layer of skin) and the dermis (or deeper layers of skin), where collagen, elastin, and other essential proteins are usually found. The cells of our body absorb and transform the photons of red-light into energy, which can then be used to increase the synthesis of collagen, elastin, and adenosine triphosphate (ATP). This allows the cells to consume more energy and enhances the skin's oxygenation and circulation while also repairing damaged tissue. This subsequently results in better skin texture due to increased collagen synthesis; additionally, red-light can reduce inflammation and germs, as well as treating precancerous lesions.

It is hypothesized that red-light works by causing a metabolic reaction in cells that enhances the mitochondria, which are the cell's powerhouse and produce most of the cell's energy. Additionally, ATP (adenosine triphosphate) is the energy-carrying chemical found in the cells of all living organisms. RLT improves mitochondrial activity, allowing cells to produce more ATP. Ultimately, this helps the cells work more efficiently, renew themselves, and repair damage with incredible energy.

RLT differs from laser therapy and intense pulsed light (IPL) therapy since this does not damage the skin's surface. Laser and pulsed light treatments induce tissue healing by controlled damage to the skin's outer layer. By promoting skin regeneration immediately, RLT avoids this arduous process. RLT's light penetrates the skin about 5 mm beneath the surface.

Red Light Therapy and Nerve Damage

Low-Level Laser Therapy (LLLT) is a new therapeutic option for neuropathic pain management, operating by inducing biochemical changes in cells. Infrared light treatment improves blood flow, temporarily relieves pain, and supplies oxygen and nutrients to the neurons; it also promotes blood flow to the extremities, which is critical in diabetic peripheral neuropathy. Diabetic neuropathy treatment aims to slow the development of diabetes, relieve pain, control muscular weakness, and regain function and mobility. Patients who use light therapy as a non-invasive option have reported feeling better after utilizing this modality.

Yamany *et al.* performed a case-controlled study on patients with painful diabetic neuropathy and found a substantial reduction in neuropathic pain after four weeks of treatment with scanning helium-neon infrared light therapy. A review conducted by Anju *et al.* showed the effectiveness of LLLT for patients with painful diabetic peripheral neuropathy.

LLLT results in photochemical reactions inside cells and higher oxygen consumption by accelerating the pace of redox reactions, enhancing ATP (adenosine triphosphate) synthesis, and increasing the production of anti-inflammatory cytokines in patients with diabetic neuropathy to relieve their symptoms.

Can Red Light Therapy Help a Person Regenerate Sensory Perception?

Until the invention of LLLT, it was thought that a diabetic patient's loss of feeling in their feet and legs was permanent and unstoppable. Anti-inflammatory medications, which block pain pathways, are still prescribed today as a first recourse. One of the most promising developments in the therapy of peripheral neuropathy is near infrared light (NIR). NIR has bio-stimulating actions on nerve cells that are beneficial for both inflammatory and neuropathic pain, making it a viable treatment option.

Recently, photo-biomodulation using red to near-infrared light-emitting diodes (LEDs) has been shown to speed up wound healing, reduce optic nerve degeneration, and stimulate tissue development. Near-infrared light treatment can successfully relieve neuropathic pain while encouraging the repair of injured nerve cells. Fibroblasts are essential for nerve regeneration, and near-infrared light stimulates their development.

According to the research, NIR light is an antioxidant and lowers inflammation, promoting neuron regeneration. Oxidative stress causes inflammation, which disrupts neuron function. Additionally, nitric oxide (NO) generation is boosted by NIR light treatment. NO aids in vasodilation or relaxing the inner muscles of blood vessels. Vasodilation is the widening of blood vessels, improving circulation and making more nutrients and oxygen available to all regions of the body.

Perhaps most importantly, LLLT helps nerve regeneration by releasing growth factors, such as nerve growth factor (NGF), brain-derived neurotrophic factor (BDNF), ciliary neurotrophic factors, essential fibroblast growth factors, and other neurotrophic factors. Photo-biomodulation

> I have felt better after receiving my Red-Light therapy for my neuropathy. The cold/numb feeling in my feet is almost gone. I can stand and walk for longer periods of time.
>
> ~ Ann A

increases the electrical properties of tissue, reduces pain, and promotes the development of vascular tissues. That is how this approach can help to reduce numbness, pain, and dysfunction associated with nerve damage and accelerate the nerve regeneration process.

How Long Does It Take For Red-Light Therapy to Have a Positive Effect on the Nervous System?

Although red-light therapy, as with many other healthcare strategies, may not provide an immediately identifiable benefit, it is essential to know that positive effects *are* taking place. For some people red light therapy can take up to four months to show visible, significant results, and it can be helpful to think of red-light treatment as "cellular exercise." Red-light treatment improves the cells' capacity to create energy, in the same way that weightlifting builds muscle and cardio exercise strengthens the heart and lungs. One wouldn't expect to see significant improvements in the body immediately after just a couple of visits to the gym. Similarly, it pays to be patient with the cells; some may notice faster improvements than others, just as each person responds differently to exercise.

As red-light therapy acts on a cellular level, the most significant results of the treatment emerge over time. Like all other cells in the body, nerve cells require time to repair or regenerate damage, and results are based on the degree of severity and extent of the nerve damage.

Consistency is essential for effective results with red light therapy; however, most people experience benefits after a few months of doing 10 to 20 minutes daily, three to five times a week. The wavelength of infrared light begins permeating the skin up to 2.36 inches after a 20-

minute NIR light treatment session. This improves blood flow, which helps alleviate neuropathic pain and inflammation in the feet by supplying oxygen, proteins, and minerals.

The procedure of RLT is entirely natural. Unlike UV radiation from the sun, it exposes the skin to acceptable quantities of light. As a result, there is almost no chance of side effects when receiving RLT. However, tissue and cell damage might occur if a practitioner has less experience or if a patient is exposed to too intense a treatment. Misusing products for home use can cause skin injury, burns, or harm to exposed eyes.

Bjordal *et al.* calculated that LLLT could decrease pain levels by 26.4% over four weeks of treatment in patients with diabetic neuropathy. Neurotransmissions found in the spinal cord's dorsal horn are required to perceive this pain, and this therapy blocks the abnormal activity of the affected nerves, thereby relieving pain. RLT is typically safe and may be a promising treatment choice for patients with diabetic peripheral neuropathy.

Additional Benefits of LED Therapy

- Can improve acne. RLT can reduce redness

and the skin's oil production, decreasing the presence of bacteria.

- Promotes anti-aging. RLT promotes the synthesis of collagen, elastin, and hyaluronic acid in the skin.
- Aids in wound healing. RLT improves circulation, oxygenation, and blood flow to the injured area.
- Treats cold sores. RLT can stimulate an immune response against infections caused by the herpes virus, enhancing the production of anti-inflammatory cytokines and thereby healing the cold sore.

CHAPTER 8

PULSED ELECTRO-MAGNETIC FIELD THERAPY

P ulsed electro-magnetic field (PEMF) therapy utilizes a specific technology to exercise and stimulate cells, thereby helping to resolve dysfunction at a cellular level and enhancing overall well- being. The use of PEMF therapy dates as far back to 2000 BCE, when the use of magnetic stones was described in the book "The Yellow Emperor's Book of Internal Medicine."

How Does Pulsed Electromagnetic Field Therapy Work?

You could view PEMF therapy as a battery charger for your cells. A healthy cell has a voltage of around -20 to -25 millivolts. When this voltage falls below -15 millivolts, a person can become sick. Once the voltage of the cells drops below this level, they cannot heal and become dysfunctional.

PEMF therapy induces a mild electromagnetic current into these damaged cells, which stops or slows the release of inflammatory and pain mediators. This increased blood flow to the cells restores regular interaction between them. As the inflammation decreases, there is also a reduction in pain, an increase in energy, and faster healing of tissues.

More than 2,000 clinical studies have evaluated the positive effects of pulsed electromagnetic field therapy on the body. These studies have covered issues related to arthritis, blood circulation, cell regeneration, pain, and wound healing on the skin. Graak *et al.* used PEMF on diabetic neuropathy subjects and found that it significantly reduced pain and improved other markers of neuropathy.

Understanding the Action of PEMF

Various distinct published neurological and physiological studies demonstrate that pulsed electromagnetic fields stimulate the mitochondria of cells, thus creating an increase in cellular respiration, which provides more energy in the form of adenosine triphosphate (ATP) with reduced oxidation waste. After several weeks of PEMF, the cells were so detoxified and produced such high ATP levels that they reverted from a mature or adult cell stage to the developmental stage, DNA signature of a young person.

Understanding the Benefits of Pulsed Electromagnetic Field Therapy

Using PEMF regularly can promote various healing mechanisms and has substantially beneficial neurological, psychological, and neuroendocrine effects. It can also enhance nerve, tissue, and bone regeneration. Various clinical studies have demonstrated that PEMF therapy is capable of the following:

- Increasing blood circulation
- Reducing inflammation
- Enhancing the function of the muscles
- Accelerating healing of the bones
- Improving oxygenation of the blood
- Decreasing the adverse effects of stress

According to a study published in the journal *Physical Therapy in Sports*,(Jeon) applying PEMF was beneficial in decreasing the physiological symptoms associated with delayed onset muscle soreness, including an improvement in the recovery of muscle soreness. Pulsed electromagnetic field therapy can be done on almost any person.

Research with PEMF has proven to be safe and without any unexpected or expected adverse reactions connected to its use. However, mild, and temporary discomfort may occur for some people, especially when initiating treatment. Some soft and temporary adverse reactions may happen in people with electromagnetic hypersensitivity, yet the therapy is usually not discontinued in such situations. Any issues tend to resolve when the treatment is slightly adjusted.

PEMF therapy must not be used over specific implanted electrical devices, such as pacemakers, cochlear implants, and intrathecal pumps; this precaution is essential to ensure that the performance of these embedded devices is not affected by the magnetic field. Moreover, PEMF must also not be performed on pregnant patients or open wounds that are bleeding (or post-operative wounds).

Furthermore, applicators should not be placed over the body's sensitive organs, such as the eyes, brain, or prostate gland. Studies have found that placing applicators over the heart may improve congestive heart failure, but this should be done with caution and only by a trained professional.

Conditions Treated by PEMF Therapy

Since a cellular reaction occurs in each part of the body, applying a magnetic field is not specific to any condition. Hence, PEMF therapy may be used to treat multiple conditions.

For Nerve Regeneration

The institutions and professionals who aim to treat neurodegenerative diseases include neurologists, chiropractors, and physical therapists, as well as regenerative medicine practitioners, orthopedists, rehabilitation centers, and senior care centers. Wellness centers would find PEMF therapy among the some of the best treatments to be used for their client's needs. People suffering from various neurological diseases, such as back pain, sciatica, ruptured or herniated discs, cervical pain, arthritis, strokes, multiple sclerosis, Alzheimer's disease, and Parkinson's disease, can benefit tremendously from PEMF.

PEMF therapy promotes symptoms of nerve regeneration, such as a slight increase in pain initially and then rapid pain relief in the long term for chronic pain conditions.

For Pain Management

PEMF therapy may accelerate the healing process, reducing the pain and making movement easier.

For Injury, Healing, and Recovery

Regular use of PEMF therapy allows the muscles to work for a longer duration and to recover more quickly. PEMF therapy stimulates the production of energy in the muscles and increases cell power by up to 500%.

PEMF therapy can increase oxygen uptake into muscles by a minimum of 1%, considerably improving performance and endurance. Moreover, pulsed electromagnetic field therapy enhances the growth of blood vessels, increasing circulation and helping tissues get their needed nutrients while removing generated waste products.

If you are a casual exerciser, you may experience less tenderness and pain post-exercise when using PEMF. If you are a competitive athlete, the recovery time between training can be shortened, and your training may be more effective. Furthermore, in general, this implies that a healthier internal environment is created in the body, making it less prone to injury.

For Stress Reduction

It has been demonstrated in various studies that the regular use of PEMF therapy changes the body's stress responses by acting directly on the significant related elements, such as the nervous and endocrine systems, and the organs or cells of the body.

For Better Sleep

PEMF therapy may help improve the quality of your sleep, as well as aid in relaxation and sustaining a sound sleep throughout the night. Pulsed electromagnetic field therapy helps to relax both the body and the mind. It promotes the release of two hormones - human growth hormone and melatonin - which are vital for deep sleep and longevity. Melatonin is one of the most crucial hormones for sleep and anti-aging. The production of melatonin is stimulated by PEMF therapy in the body's pineal gland.

> *The PEMF at Dr. Chaney's office really does the trick to get me recharged and tackle my week. You can feel it working through the whole body. I get more energy to take on my chores and sleep better.*
>
> ~ Kendal

For Mental Focus

PEMF therapy programs promote an alpha state of mind - an awakened but relaxed state. During this state, the mind can learn and retain much more information without having to review it continuously. Another PEMF therapy program induces beta brain waves, during which the ability to multitask, problem-solve, and process data is increased. This can allow you to have fewer distractions, more mental focus, and become highly productive.

Understanding the Pulsed Electromagnetic Field Therapy Device and How Its Mechanism Works

To apply pulsed electromagnetic field therapy, an electric current is passed through a copper coil, giving rise to a magnetic field. This is assimilated into various devices, the most often used and most effective one being the full- body therapy mat. You must either lie down on the mat or place the applicator onto the targeted area that requires treatment. The PEMF will then enter the body and target cells, muscle tissue, and bones.

PEMF is a safe and natural treatment for neuropathic pain, as it relieves pain by reducing inflammation and improving blood circulation. Regular PEMF therapy can also delay the progression of diabetic neuropathy.

According to research, a minimum of 12 minutes per day of PEMF therapy was used for diabetic neuropathy and resulted in improved pain, sensation, and increased strength in the muscles of 85% of patients compared to control groups. PEMF therapy is not new; it has been effectively and safely used across Europe and America for over five decades.

CHAPTER 9

THE POWER OF VIBRATION THERAPY

W hole-body vibration (WBV) therapy was initially developed for athletes to improve the effectiveness of their training. Vibration platforms would be included in some regular conditioning and gym exercises such as squats, press- ups, and step-ups. The therapy is undertaken by standing, sitting, lying, or doing exercises on specifically designed equipment that oscillates, generally in a horizontal plane, at relatively high frequencies.

The plates vibrate, sending mechanical vibrations through your body, somewhere between 20 and 60 times per second (this can be adjusted). This requires your muscles to contract and relax between 20 and 60 times per second to stabilize your body. These muscular contractions are supposed to make you build muscle, lose fat, become stronger, as well as improve circulation.

Vibration signals are transmitted into one's skin, muscle tissue, and tendons to stimulate more powerful muscular contractions. This can assist with increased muscle strength, coordination, and balance over time. With this, improved control of blood sugar levels is created, thanks to a greater ability to burn energy due to the augmented level of muscular mass. Current theory also suggests that bone cells are sensitive to this vibration and respond by increasing bone density. This has a further impact on better sugar control.

WBV for Neuropathy

WBV has been used in patients with neurological or musculoskeletal disorders as a new and effective intervention method to improve physical function. Recently, WBV has been applied to enhance the strength and balance of diabetic patients. WBV can be an effective and relatively inexpensive therapeutic modality compared to prescription drugs, in treating patients with painful diabetic neuropathy.

Recent research has demonstrated the positive impact WBV can have on balance in patients with peripheral neuropathy, and the application of WBV in the treatment of diabetic peripheral neuropathy has shown to be multifactorial. Improving distal extremity strength will likely improve balance control, an important consequence of peripheral neuropathy.

Indeed gait, pain intensity and quality of life were all noted improvements in patients with diabetic neuropathy. With improved gait, the risk of serious injury from falling is reduced. Additionally, Kessler *et al.* performed a WBV study on patients with diabetic peripheral neuropathy. The participants had three WBV session per week, with at least on day in between sessions, 12 min/session (four bouts of 3 min) for four weeks. The control group received sham treatment. The WBV group had significant improvement in pain, balance, and quality of life scores, compared to the control group. Furthermore, WBV participants reported reduced diabetic PN-related pain for 1 to 5 weeks after treatment.

What is the Science Behind WBV?

WBV works very similarly to the knee-jerk reflex; the same reflex that is triggered when you sit on an exam table in your doctor's office and the doctor taps your kneecap. You have no control over your lower leg motion. When muscles are activated via a "stretch reflex," your body has no choice but to react. WBV technology exploits this fact by using an external stimulus, the vibrating platform. You then load a muscle or muscle group in line with the direction of the vibration by assuming various positions, like some yoga poses. Your muscles respond to the vibration as compensation, with a brief reflex contraction, of virtually all muscle fibers of that specific muscle.

WBV and exercise reduced insulin levels by similar amounts in the mice tested and increased their responsiveness to insulin. In patients who are obese or have type 2 diabetes, fat often accumulates in the liver which can lead to organ malfunction and even death. But the mice that worked out on the treadmill or lived in the vibrating cages carried about one-third as much fat in the liver as the control group.

The vibrations cause the muscles of the body to contract and relax several times a second. WBV machines can be found at sports rehabilitation centers and offices of physical therapists. Smaller machines that you stand on can be purchased for home use. On machines with large platforms, it is possible to do simple exercises, like squats and lunges, to enhance fitness results. Many people find it challenging to exercise regularly, a contributing factor to the obesity and diabetic epidemic. These disorders can increase the risk of bone fractures, and physical activity can help to decrease those risks and reduce the adverse metabolic effects of each condition.

WBV training is suitable for both beginners and advanced patients. It is not difficult and can be used for beginner workouts and by senior citizens. Yet, more advanced patients can increase the difficulty and make it more challenging. Athletes have used whole-body vibration training for years as a tool to improve their strength, flexibility, and endurance.

When you use a WBV platform for training, rehabilitation, or therapy, you're getting an unbelievable workout. All the exercises are done either standing, sitting, or lying down. Due to the frequency of the platform movement, in just 10 minutes using a WBV machine, you can get the equivalent of 60 minutes of conventional exercise at a gym.

The benefits of WBV training are considerable, evidenced by its acceptance by major medical, rehabilitation, and therapeutic centers across the country. The health benefits are multifold, and results can be achieved easily. WBV can enhance your general well-being and quality of life regardless of age, medical, neurological, or physical condition. WBV training is not difficult, but it can be challenging — however, the degree of difficulty is entirely up to you.

How Long Does It Take to See Results with Whole Body Vibration?

Each session only takes between 10 to15 minutes to complete. Excellent results are seen to occur from 6 weeks of exercising, at least twice a week. Imagine performing 10,000 muscle contractions in one session. 10 minutes is all the time it takes to quickly warm up your entire body, exercise the areas you want to improve, and then cool down.

What Does Whole Body Vibration Do to the Brain?

No, the WBV machine does not rattle, damage, or harm the brain. Your brain will encounter more jarring from a bicycle ride or a one-mile jog, than from the WBV machine. What really happens is that the movement, during vibration plate exercises, causes the brain to communicate messages to the muscles, to contract and maintain equilibrium effectively, creating a muscle-toning and therapeutic isometric workout. As the muscles contract, they are strengthening as well as causing an increase in circulation, which brings nutrients to the muscles. The itching sensation often felt on the equipment is an indication of improved blood flow to the skin.

Additional Benefits of Whole Body Vibration

During WBV Machine training, almost 100% of the muscle fibers are utilized, which improves blood circulation, lymphatic drainage, and metabolism.

> *I was having issues with muscle and balance loss on the right side of my body. Dr. Steph gave me great training workouts on the vibration plate in the office. I immediately started to feel the difference. I have regained the ability to squeeze certain muscles on the right side as well. I once thought my bed was not level and complained to my husband. Well, it was just me, not anymore!*
>
> *~ KJ*

A WVB machine stimulates the muscles to pump blood into the smallest capillaries of the body, allowing the cells to receive fuel more rapidly and causing waste products to be disposed of much faster. Also, by enhancing your local circulation, they help to build a better immune system.

The following are some of the major benefits of WBV.

Muscular Strength

There is an increase in muscle growth when performing isometric exercises on the vibration machine. Everyone, including seniors, can benefit greatly from this. If you have knee osteoarthritis, you may increase your muscle strength by doing exercise positions such as lunges, dips, and squats for 60 to 90 seconds as little as three times per week, the best you can.

Special Needs

For people with various disabilities who are unable to undergo regular strength training exercises, whole-body vibration can offer a great deal of benefits. They can strengthen their muscles with little impact on their joints or stress on their cardiovascular system. People who have multiple sclerosis or suffer from Parkinson's disease can also take advantage of this machine to increase strength and stability, balance, and flexibility. Even the very elderly can use and benefit from vibration exercise training.

Increased Flexibility

Vibration training increases flexibility. Synovial fluid is released into the joints within 90 seconds, resulting in lubrication that enhances movement. Also, the stiff muscles resulting from stiff joints are relaxed and loosened up to move more freely. As the circulation pumps oxygenation into the damaged joints, healing can take place. That is why there are several ways in which whole-body vibration increases flexibility, range of motion, and decreases joint pain. Osteoarthritis is one of the conditions that can greatly benefit.

Increased Bone Density

Vibration machines increase bone mineral density, for stronger bones. Improved bone density can stave off osteoporosis, a major concern for women. Also, for older individuals, increased mineral density can prevent bones from breaking if they incur a fall.

Weight Loss and Toning

These machines increase metabolism to help burn more fat while simultaneously strengthening muscles to tone and tighten. The oscillation gets your heart rate up, so you burn more fat at a higher rate. In addition, the vibration waves stimulate muscles to lengthen them and make them taut. And if you perform exercises or vary your stance, you can target specific or stubborn areas for spot training. In this way, you can sculpt the body as you lose weight which may prevent sagging or stretched skin.

Recovery

Muscle recovery is another benefit of the whole-body vibration machine. Exercisers can recover from intense physical workout by using the machine afterwards, to prevent stiffness and soreness the next day. A relaxing way to massage those tired leg muscles after a long period of standing or sitting is to lay on the floor and rest one's calves, right on the rapidly moving platform.

Health and Anti-Aging

Vibration exercises greatly increase lymphatic drainage, resulting in toxins being cleansed from the body. Blood circulation is increased by rapid muscle contractions, thereby increasing oxygenation to all the cells, which aids in repair and regeneration of damaged cells. Oxygenation plays a significant role in the prevention of disease and aging.

Therapy

WBV results in elevated HGH (human growth

hormone) levels. Suppose you have undergone surgery or suffered an injury; healing can then be enhanced through these elevated levels. Athletic injuries are also treated with sports massage by using the vibration machine. WBV also makes neuromuscular reduction possible in various situations such as stroke and multiple sclerosis.

CHAPTER 10

NEURAL ELECTRICAL THERAPY

O xygen deficiency may very well be responsible for the physical atrophy of nerve cells. When nerve cells waste away, the space between cells, called the synaptic junction, widens. A wider space prevents normal-intensity electrical impulses from jumping the synaptic junction. Neuropathy can be the result of this condition.

Neural electrical therapy is a technology designed to circumvent this gap by waking up dormant nerve cells, relaxing atrophied nerve cells, and restoring normal plus/minus polarity along the nerve axons and dendrites. It is effective for the hands, knees, elbows, back, feet, and legs. This specialized unit can produce a dramatic improve-ment in the reduction of painful symptoms; an electronic device used in the privacy of your home and fully registered by the FDA.

I feel better after my Tesla treatments [neural electrical therapy]. I can open and close my right hand better.

~ Mr Perry

Please note that it is extremely dangerous to use a traditional transcutaneous electrical nerve stimulation (TENS) or electrical muscle stimulation (EMS) device to treat neuropathy, as it can overload the nerves and cause permanent damage. The Rebuilder®, a neural electrical therapy device, however, sends a very specific signal to your feet, hands, and legs that travels up and down and is an exact duplicate of an average nerve signal.

Think of it like this.... When you were young, on occasion you probably sat with your leg under your buttocks, with your leg then "falling asleep." It tingled and felt numb. So, what did you naturally do? You simply moved your leg (stopping the cause), stomped your foot on the ground, and the feeling in your leg returned. This worked as you sent a much larger, but normal, nerve impulse up your leg to the nerve roots of your lower back. That is exactly how the Rebuilder® works.

The device is a small, hand-held, battery-powered

nerve stimulator that sends a comfortable electronic impulse to your feet and legs. It requires a 30-minute treatment window in which the patient applies a conductive gel to each of the signal pads. The pads are then placed on the soles of the feet, the palms of the hands, and on the lower back or shoulders as needed. Rebuilder® senses different wave forms, and thus knows what area of the body is being treated. This feature is not found in other devices.

The technology accomplishes various functions in a simple-to-use home care system that is not only effective in helping relieve many of the symptoms of neuropathy and chronic pain, but also in limiting its progression. Additionally, it can cause regression of pain, burning, and numbness. When the device's electrical signals stimulate the leg muscles, causing them to contract, this "venous muscle pump" moves the mineral-rich blood out to the muscles and nerves. Osmotic pressure and the ionic tension from the signals of Rebuilder® successfully bridge the gaps, carrying these necessary minerals into the synaptic junctions between nerve cells. This helps restore the conductivity that is typically lost with neuropathy.

How Does Rebuilder® Work?

The technology works by sending its healing signals to your feet, hands, or back — small conductive rubber signal pads are placed on your skin. Then, you sit back and relax for your treatment. This excellent device uses a tiny electrical signal to wake up nerves that are temporarily dormant, or asleep. These signals mimic your natural nerve signals but are stronger. They travel from one foot, up the leg, across the synaptic junctions and nerve roots in your lower back, and down to the other foot. It then reverses polarity and travels back to the original foot. This "back-and-forth" action effectively treats the nerves of both legs and feet.

At the same time, your calf muscles are contracting and relaxing, as they would naturally do during a regular activity, like walking. An additional benefit results from the brain releasing endorphins, a strong pain reliever that travels in the bloodstream to all parts of the body. These natural pain relievers are known to relieve depression and physical pain without any adverse side effects. The Rebuilder® opens the nerve paths, re-educating them to transmit normal nerve signals to the brain. The resulting increased blood flow results in a therapeutic healing process, not a temporary fix.

Imagine no side effects, walking pain-free, no fear of stumbling, sleeping through the night, and feeling the carpet and grass under your feet! The device can give you these results, along with the benefits of reducing or stopping the need for drugs and pain medications. It can help relieve pain, numbness, and restore your mobility.

Three-Level Therapy

The therapy works simultaneously on three separate levels: stimulation of the nerves, stimulation of the muscles, combined electrostimulation.

The first signal is designed to stimulate the nerves by sending an electrical impulse with a very narrow waveform and a relatively high transient voltage, 40 to 90 volts AC. The resulting current is minuscule and much lower than what is commonly found with traditional TENS devices. A larger-than-normal signal must be used due to the widening gap between the nerve cells and the loss of much of the conductivity in the synaptic junction fluid due to demineralization. The nerve-stimulating signal of Rebuilder® is many times stronger than the normal afferent and efferent signals; therefore, it can effectively complete the circuit.

This stimulates the nerves, causing them to re-establish their normal metabolic function. This signal, crossing the synaptic junctions, also re-polarizes the junctions, causing them to be receptive and reabsorb minerals, thus improving conductivity.

The second signal stimulates the muscles with a different, wider waveform and a larger subthreshold amount of current under the curve and a much smaller voltage (5 to 20 AC). Muscles are most responsive to this waveform. This signal causes the muscles of the feet, calves, thighs, and buttocks to contract and relax harmoniously with the therapy's signal. It overcomes any residual inflammatory resistance to blood flow; the device's proprietary signal also has specific characteristics that cause a complete relaxation of the muscles' fast and slow twitch cells between each contraction stimulus.

The third signal is combined electrostimulation. This twin electrical signal (one to stimulate the nerve cells and the other to trigger muscle cells) is pulsed on and off at the frequency of 7.83 cycles per second. One postulation for this sensitivity is that the electrical potential between

Earth's atmosphere and Earth's surface is also approximately 7.83 Hz. Simultaneously stimulating the muscles of the feet, calves, thighs, and buttocks, Rebuilder® evokes complete relaxation between each contraction stimulus. This increases the flow of oxygen- rich blood to the synaptic junctions, affording effective and efficient conduction of nerve signals - combined electro-stimulation uses twin electrical signals to stimulate the nerves and muscle cells.

Using this signal frequency, the body not only responds favorably but the brain is induced to release large amounts of endorphins, producing a sense of well-being, and reducing anxiety, as well as physical and emotional trauma. Endorphins, the internal analgesics, are as powerful as and chemically related to morphine, but without any negative side effects. They are created and modulated by the body's chemistry. The impact of this endorphin release is a generalized sense of well-being, a reduction in pain and anxiety levels elsewhere in the body, and even a reduction in emotional pain. Reduction of pain will lead to improvement in patient compliance and quality of life.

Additionally, the therapy features a simultaneous weighted DC signal designed to stabilize the trigger threshold that regulates the sensitivity of the nerve cell. By sending this constant DC signal, the resting potential is held at a fixed voltage long enough for the cell to stabilize itself and regain control.

Benefits of Using Rebuilder®

The Rebuilder® is a great adjunct therapy for neuropathy. Through its actions, healing of damaged nerves can begin, and neuropathic pain can be alleviated. Following are the mechanisms by which the neuropathic patient can benefit.

- Stimulates the leg muscles to contract and relax, increasing blood velocity and volume with fresh blood to the nerves and muscles.
- Stimulates all the afferent and efferent nerves in the lower extremities, with a signal larger than average, to re- establish the pathways for subsequent normal signals to follow.
- Draws axon and dendrite nerve endings closer together to facilitate proper nerve transmission.
- Causes the brain to release endorphins that reduce global pain and anxiety.
- Promotes the healing of non-plantar surface diabetic skin ulcers and sprains.

- Increases muscle strength for safe, pain-free walking.
- Reduces edema, as muscle contractions encourage lymphatic drainage and movement to the proper nodes.

How Long Does It Take to Begin Seeing Benefits
with Rebuilder® Therapy?

As with any treatment, results vary from individual to individual. Some clients report immediate results, while others report positive results after as much as five to seven months. Response to treatment is influenced by many factors, such as whether the individual is dealing with multiple medical conditions in addition to the number and classes of prescription drugs they may be taking. It has been our experience, however, that individuals who are persistent in following their treatment regimen will ultimately gain an improvement in their condition.

Finally, Rebuilder® treatment for nerve pain is safe, effective, without side effects, and very easy to use. You can experience immediate, total relief from your symptoms during your first 30-minute treatment at home. After your 30-minute treatment, you can experience a 50% to 70%

reduction in your symptoms for 3 to 4 hours. When used before bedtime, it can help you fall asleep faster and sleep comfortably throughout the night.

> *The Rebuilder machine took away the numbness in my feet. Now I can ride my bicycle again!*
>
> ~ Tom R

What Are the Contraindications Associated with Rebuilder® Therapy?

There are no negative side effects when using Rebuilder® according to the directions. However, we have had reports of sore or cramping calf muscles resulting from using it at too high a setting for a sustained period, much like exercising too much, too quickly. Initially use the Rebuilder® at a low setting, thereby allowing the feet and legs time to adjust to the stimulation.

On rare occasions an individual may experience headache or nausea. This infrequent reaction can happen due to an adrenaline rush for users who harbor a latent, general fear of electricity. That subconscious fear can produce adrenaline, which in turn produces temporary headaches or nausea. However, there are positive side effects of using the unit.

As a result of nerve stimulation, the brain releases endorphins which help relax muscles and reduce pain in other parts of the body. Our system also helps to increase mobility by building muscle mass, improving leg strength, and promoting better balance. In addition, many clients also report experiencing a better night's rest and a reduction in the need for pain medications.

Rebuilder® Versus TENS Unit

Rebuilder® neuropathy therapy is completely different from any other treatment system offered anywhere in the world to treat the painful symptoms of nerve pain. The device's built-in microprocessor measures several physiological functions of your nerves, and automatically adjusts itself to your specific therapeutic needs, beginning with the first healing signal. While sitting in your chair or bed, this signal travels automatically from one foot, up the leg, across the nerve roots in the lower back, and then down the other leg, to the other foot.

The device impulse utilizes tiny amounts of current under the curve and a high transient voltage of 40 to 90 volts. The resultant current is below that commonly produced by traditional TENS units. The device delivers a second, simultaneous, lower voltage (5-20 volts), wider waveform signal designed to stimulate muscle tissue. This signal causes the muscles of the feet, calves, thighs, and buttocks to intermittently contract and relax. Stimulating the venous muscle pump to empty veins, thus allowing whatever arterial pressure is present to fill the vacated veins quickly. This enhances local blood flow.

Additionally, Rebuilder® utilizes multiple bio-feedback loops that enable the device to measure and analyze nerve function before, during, and after the treatment. This means that every 0.12 seconds, Rebuilder® is responding to your physiological status, creating, and delivering a unique signal.

As for other traditional TENS units, it is extremely dangerous to use a common TENS or EMS device to treat neuropathy, as it can overload the nerves causing permanent damage. This technology sends a specific signal to your feet, hands, and legs that travels up and down and is an exact duplicate of a normal nerve signal. Rather than simply numbing your nerves, like drugs or other

TENS-like devices, Rebuilder® can calm down your overactive nerves and wake up your underactive nerves. Also, the device's healing signals include electronic muscle stimulation which automatically strengthens nearby calf muscles (or arm muscles, when used for hand pain), and increases local blood flow to enhance permanent healing.

CHAPTER 11

PHASES OF HEALING

T his chapter is dedicated to describing specific phases of healing to better explain how increasing your strength, health, and longevity can be approached. First, let us clarify. Chiropractic care, as with all natural healing approaches, is not a quick fix or an overnight miracle. Suppose your system is currently out of balance; it is certain that other issues have been present for a long time, leading to the development of any unhealthy condition you are presently experiencing. The good news is that it will not necessarily take years to regain your health, however, it may take some time and dedication on your part.

1 - The Intense Inflammatory Phase

This is a phase in which people are encouraged to

pay more attention to their health and to seek expert help. Most pain experienced during this phase is characterized by strong discomfort.

At this stage, patients often come to see the chiropractor with complaints of severe pain or signs of pronounced discomforts, such as swelling, soreness, aches, stiffness, difficulty sitting or walking, or a loss of balance. Often, patients at this stage do not visit us because they want to improve their health but because they are fed up with the pain or discomfort. Their main concern is reducing their pain and seeking immediate relief — not the underlying mechanics that may be the cause of their issue.

It must be emphasized that the body does not arrive at such a stage overnight; it took *years* to reach such a painful state — years of mishandling and inappropriate movements, stress, a poor diet, mismanagement, and strain. Therefore, healing at this initial stage may also require time, and you might have to visit a chiropractor's office once or twice a week for a while. Although this may sound exaggerated to the average person seeking a quick fix, it is a small investment for your long-term health.

Please note that treatment can vary in frequency and need based on the following factors:

- Sex,
- Age,
- Height,
- Weight,
- The length of time you have been suffering from the health issue,
- The degree to which you follow your physician's directions,
- The amount of pain you can tolerate,
- Other health problems you are experiencing.

At the initial consultation, the chiropractor will assess all the above parameters, as well as any other relevant aspects or problems, to design a personalized plan for your care. Your personal needs and challenges are considered. Thus, any chiropractic approach is tailored to you, rather than a one-size-fits-all approach.

Chiropractic methods are not painful by nature. What can trigger any sensation of pain is your body's reaction to the state of sore tissue and muscles, or pinched nerves, signaling pain throughout the body when the chiropractor works on them. If your body is inflamed, painful, or other health-related issues for an extended period, it may be more sensitive to pain than a normal, healthy body.

2 - The Restorative and Corrective Phase

During this phase, your pain and discomfort begin to subside and become more tolerable. You may not feel as though you are progressing at lightning speeds, but you should experience much less discomfort and have a more cheerful outlook toward your health. We rely on this phase to rehabilitate strength and integrity, and to stabilize the patient on their road to full recovery. This is an excellent stage as the patient begins to experience positive change. Energy levels increase, discomfort is minimized, and some range of motion is restored. As pain "eats" away vast amounts of energy, the reduction of pain and the boost in energy levels can be remarkable!

However, there is one aspect that we need to pay extra attention to during this phase: avoiding pushing or forcing the body too much. When most people begin to feel better under treatment, they might mistakenly think they are able to do more than they really can. The dilemma is pushing oneself too hard, too early, and causing strain or inappropriate stress, which can result in renewed damage or setbacks.

During this phase, our chiropractic aim focuses on boosting spinal mobility so that healthy physiological functions are restored to your spine and nerves, which connect all parts of your body. You may still have to visit your chiropractor once a week, but it all depends on the intensity of your condition.

Keep in mind that this corrective stage is not usually brief, and that other parameters and factors affect the speed of healing. The following things can affect treatment and slow progress, such as:

- Poor diet or lack of nutrition,
- Smoking,
- Stress,
- Improper ergonomics,
- A negative mindset.

3 – The Maintenance Phase

We love having patients at this specific stage visit us! Arriving at this stage means that they have followed the treatment directions and are doing what they can to restore their health and well-being. At this stage, pain is minimal, controlled, and managed at least. Once the body achieves a state of *good* health, it is necessary to maintain it. Fortunately, keeping your body healthy is much easier at this phase. Remember, a state of perfect health does not just imply a lack of pain and disease, it is a state of optimal physical, mental, and personal well- being.

When your body is in optimal health, not only do you benefit from better physical performance but also faster recovery time if any accidents should occur. Consider children and the rate they often recover from injuries. This is because our system is designed to recover and restore health quickly from a very young age. As we grow older, the rate of recovery deteriorates, and we are often less resistant and less able to fight off health issues. It comes down to lifelong habits and health patterns. This is where people may experience a certain degree of discomfort as they transition to a healthier diet, exercise more, and build a positive, stress-free mindset.

Often, the excuses that stand in the way at this point are classic ones, such as a lack of sufficient time to exercise, prepare healthy food, or ensure sound sleep. There should always be time to decide what is essential for a better quality of life and make that your priority. It would be best if you took care of your health, in your own way.

Nathaniel Branden, an inspiring psychologist who has written several books on self-confidence and self-esteem, believes that the things we try to improve are those we have already realized are flawed. In contrast, the areas we neglect to work on are those we ignore, and feel are beyond our control. This also applies to our health: You must work on it every day, and you will eventually be able to efficiently work towards achieving it once you have the necessary means.

> *I had significant neuropathy including cold sensations, tingling, and numbness in both feet. My treatment has progressed to maintenance now and I am free from those symptoms 98% of the time. My neurologist told me he had nothing to help with idiopathic neuropathy other than the normal pills, so I took a chance with this integrative treatment. I am pleased with the results it has achieved for me.*
>
> *~ Mike B*

People tend to make this step overly complicated, but here are a few questions you can use to help improve your health.

- How can I enjoy eating properly today and working out?
- What foods can I eat that are healthy and delicious?
- What type of exercise or activity can I do that I would enjoy doing?
- How can I fuel my system with the right food it requires?

- Why do I have to eat better quality foods?
- Why should I exercise today?

The 9 Key Habits of Healthy Folks

Now that you are familiar with the primary phases of healing within chiropractic, we can move on to the nine essential habits that healthy people practice daily, which are vital for their health. This information may help you make better decisions regarding your health.

These nine habits will change your lifestyle one step at a time. It is essential to take a gradual and slow approach when implementing meaningful change. Otherwise, you are likely to burn out and may give up, convincing yourself that the change was a bad idea or something you did not want.

Here are the fundamental principles.

1. Water/Hydration

Drink at least eight glasses of purified water daily, as this can substantially impact the body's power to preserve health and fight off illness.

2. Eat Vegetables

Increasing your daily consumption of greens is one of the wisest nutritional choices you can make for your health.

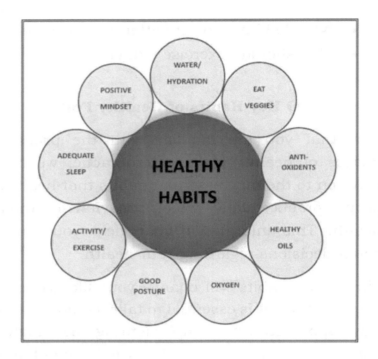

3. Remember Antioxidants

Free radicals are not only triggered by the natural aging process but also by other factors such as stress, injuries, or a poor diet containing processed and chemical-laden foods. Green vegetables, fruits, and nuts are naturally enriched with antioxidants and nutrients.

4. Healthy Oils Are a Must

An insufficient intake of essential fatty acids is linked to heart and brain problems, as well as many types of inflammatory disorders. Only certain fats and oils are healthy, including fish avocadoes and flaxseed oil.

5. Proper Oxygenation

Practice mindful, deep breathing methods supported by cardio exercise.

6. A Good Posture

How we stand or sit can affect how well we breathe, and a poor posture can put stress on the spinal curve, which in turn can cause problems with the nervous system.

7. Physical Activity/Exercise

Exercise and physical activity are vital to your health. Your system needs a complete cardio workout plan that activates the important muscles in your body, such as the heart. You need to challenge it so that it pumps more blood and oxygen throughout your body.

8. Adequate Sleep

Insufficient sleep is a known culprit of poor health. People who do not get enough sleep have a higher risk of suffering from the consequences of a weakened immune system.

9. Positive Mindset

It is possible to be "overly positive," but there is a

valid point to having a positive mindset. If you catch a cold, complaining and moaning about it will probably make you feel worse! However, if you try to approach it with a positive outlook and focus on getting better, instead of cursing it and paying attention to feeling ill, you may recover quicker.

If you practice these nine lifestyle habits and incorporate them into your life, it is much more likely that you will create a healthier, happier reality for yourself.

CHAPTER 12

IN CONCLUSION

O ur bodies have an incredible capacity for healing, and our nervous system is a powerful agent in keeping us healthy and functional. This book provides an accessible resource for anyone wanting to better understand the causes of neuropathy, available treatments, both traditional and holistic, and how to best manage nerve pain and reverse the debilitating effects of neuropathy. We hope we inspired you to act today.

We have covered several treatment options, from oxygen to diet and from lights to frequencies. There is something for everyone. The diabetic epidemic and rampage of chronic pain have a strong hold on our country. The modernized plight of the inflammatory syndrome and the destructive effect of sugar in our diets have effectively lowered the quality of life for too many in the United States.

Our current healthcare system is not effective in helping us live healthy and pain-free lives. The model of sick care and symptom treatment no longer serves us, and we need to educate ourselves more on the vital benefits of preventive healthcare. There is powerful knowledge about nutritious food, proper exercise, beneficial healthcare habits, and how personalized functional medicine and chiropractic care may support the body's own innate intelligence.

People used to think that if there were no major medical breakthroughs, the average life expectancy would be pretty much the same as it is now — around 75 years old. However, some of us think there is room for improvement, and that the current population estimates are too low. The demographers who conducted this research looked at deaths and illnesses in different countries around the world and found that Americans have some of the worst health outcomes in the world.

A staggering 50 million Americans suffer from chronic pain - pain that has been present for more than 12 weeks. Chronic pain is particularly common among women and elderly individuals, those who have previously held employment, recipients of public health insurance services, and rural dwellers. Eight percent of those afflicted are diagnosed with high-impact chronic pain. Chronic pain is a top cause of disability in the United States, with half of all workers reporting lower back discomfort annually. Unfortunately, current healthcare costs prevent many patients from getting sufficiently treated. Chronic pain expenses exceed that of any other health complaint. Hence, it is vital to invest more in this area for long-term positive outcomes in public health.

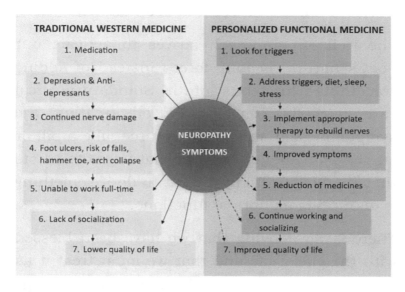

Traditional health care in the United States is often viewed as a reactive solution. If you are involved in a terrible car accident, the U.S. is the place to do it. Crisis care in America is second to none. However, if you are suffering from an infection or physical trauma, the primary function of sick care is to prevent further damage and decrease your symptoms rather than find and remove or correct the source of your clinical complaint. A more proactive approach such as holistic healthcare can help you stay healthy by making lifestyle changes which might include proper nutrition, exercise plans and alternative therapies like massage or acupuncture - all with the goal of avoiding potential issues down the line. At one extreme, we have health care that works to prevent illness and keep us well.

The wellness approach strives to activate our body's natural healing forces instead of adding something extraneous into it. Standard medical care typically concentrates on treating the symptoms from an external source, like a pill or surgery. On the other hand, naturopathy trusts that the body will know what to do if something is disrupting its normal functions.

There is no denying that we have been blessed with the gift of life and that we must treat it as such - showing gratitude for the amazing things our body does for us on a daily basis.

Innate intelligence is an intrinsic force that was ignited the moment you were conceived, and since then it has been responsible for governing your body's operations. From keeping a sound heart rhythm to promoting skin health, innate intelligence ensures that all your bodily functions remain in balance. Neuropathy is a condition that can be triggered by various things, including diabetes. It can cause damage to the peripheral nerves, which can cause pain and other symptoms. Neuropathic pain is a complex condition to manage, and current treatments often fail to provide adequate relief. There are many reasons why traditional therapies for neuropathic pain management can fail, including incorrect diagnosis, poor care of other conditions, and incorrect selection of treatment options.

Our days are filled with sugar, shallow breathing, sedentary jobs, and stress. Our nights consist of restless sleep, when we are in dire need of a deep, rejuvenating slumber. We need to do better.

Inflammatory diseases are on the rise. Chronic inflammation can have many negative consequences on the body, including developing various inflammatory disorders, which can lead to further health problems and accelerated aging. In truth, inflammation is the body's natural response to an injury. It occurs when white blood cells produce chemicals in response to the injury.

Some foods and medications increase or decrease the amount of these chemicals, and lifestyle changes can also help to reduce inflammation. Scientists are exploring the biochemical properties of pain, to discern how food can influence inflammation levels.

By comprehending the science behind inflammation, we have the power to construct a diet that lessens or eliminates our need for painkillers. Not all foods are equal when it comes to aggravating inflammation, some foods can combat it. By making simple changes in lifestyle and dietary choices, you can experience significant relief from discomfort caused by inflammation.

Rejuvenating your body through chiropractic care and an integrated approach to preventive healthcare is not a miraculous healing approach, but rather requires time and effort. Nevertheless, if you commit to the nine habits of healthy living and commit to your own state of health, you can change your life and take those first steps towards the state of wellness you desire!

It has been an honor to serve you on this journey through this book. May this book inspire you to use its principles and to restore, renew, and recreate your health to levels never before experienced. We are here for you to remind you of the incredible capacity your body has for healing.

May your life never be the same.

REFERENCES and FURTHER READING

Angelidi AM, Stambolliu E, Adamopoulou KI, Kousoulis AA. Is Atorvastatin Associated with New Onset Diabetes or Deterioration of Glycemic Control? Systematic Review Using Data from 1.9 Million Patients. Int J Endocrinol. 2018 Oct 22;2018:8380192. doi: 10.1155/2018/8380192. PMID: 30425742; PMCID: PMC6217757. https://www.ncbi.nlm.nih.gov/pmc/articles/PMC6217757/

Anju M, Ummer V S, Maiya AG, Hande M. Low level laser therapy for patients with painful diabetic peripheral neuropathy - A systematic review. Diabetes Metab Syndr. 2019 Jul-Aug;13(4):2667-2670. doi: 10.1016/j.dsx.2019.07.035. Epub 2019 Jul 13. PMID: 31405692. https://pubmed.ncbi.nlm.nih.gov/31405692/

Balducci S, Iacobellis G, Parisi L, et al. Exercise training can modify the natural history of diabetic peripheral neuropathy. J Diabetes Complications. 2006 Jul-Aug;20(4):216-23. doi: 10.1016/j.jdiacomp.2005.07.005. PMID: 16798472. https://pubmed.ncbi.nlm.nih.gov/28119442/ https://pubmed.ncbi.nlm.nih.gov/16798472/

Boegman S, Dziedzic CE. Nutrition and Supplements for Elite Open-Weight Rowing. Curr Sports Med Rep, 15(4):p 252-261, 7/8 2016. | DOI: 10.1249/JSR.0000000000000281 https://pubmed.ncbi.nlm.nih.gov/27399822/

Bjordal JM, Couppé C, Chow RT, et al. A systematic review of low level laser therapy with location-specific

doses for pain from chronic joint disorders. Aust J Physiother. 2003;49(2):107-16. doi: 10.1016/s0004-9514(14)60127-6. PMID: 12775206.
https://pubmed.ncbi.nlm.nih.gov/12775206/

Broers MC, Bunschoten C, Nieboer D, et al. Incidence and Prevalence of Chronic Inflammatory Demyelinating Polyradiculoneuropathy: A Systematic Review and Meta-Analysis. Neuroepidemiology. 2019;52(3-4):161-172. doi: 10.1159/000494291. Epub 2019 Jan 22. PMID: 30669140; PMCID: PMC6518865.
https://pubmed.ncbi.nlm.nih.gov/30669140/

Clavo B, Rodríguez-Abreu D, Galván S, et al. Long-term improvement by ozone treatment in chronic pain secondary to chemotherapy-induced peripheral neuropathy: A preliminary report. Front Physiol. 2022 Aug 30;13:935269. doi: 10.3389/fphys.2022.935269. PMID: 36111149; PMCID: PMC9468657.
https://pubmed.ncbi.nlm.nih.gov/36111149/

Esposito K, Maiorino MI, Bellastella G, et al. A journey into a Mediterranean diet and type 2 diabetes: a systematic review with meta-analyses. BMJ Open. 2015 Aug 10;5(8):e008222. doi: 10.1136/bmjopen-2015-008222. PMID: 26260349; PMCID: PMC4538272.
https://pubmed.ncbi.nlm.nih.gov/26260349/

Feldman EL, Callaghan BC, Pop-Busui R, et al. Diabetic neuropathy. Nat Rev Dis Primers. 2019 Jun 13;5(1):42. doi: 10.1038/s41572-019-0097-9. PMID: 31197183; PMCID: PMC7096070.
https://www.ncbi.nlm.nih.gov/pmc/articles/PMC7096070/

Forouzanfar F, Hosseinzadeh H. Medicinal herbs in the treatment of neuropathic pain: a review. Iran J Basic Med Sci. 2018 Apr;21(4):347-358. doi: 10.22038/IJBMS.2018.24026.6021. PMID: 29796216; PMCID: PMC5960749.
https://www.ncbi.nlm.nih.gov/pmc/articles/PMC5960749/

Graak V, Chaudhary S, Bal BS, Sandhu JS. Evaluation of the efficacy of pulsed electromagnetic field in the management of patients with diabetic polyneuropathy. Int J Diabetes Dev Ctries. 2009 Apr;29(2):56-61. doi: 10.4103/0973-3930.53121. PMID: 20142869; PMCID: PMC2812751.
https://www.ncbi.nlm.nih.gov/pmc/articles/PMC2812751/?report=reader

Harden N, Cohen M. Unmet needs in the management of neuropathic pain. J Pain Symptom Manage. 2003 May;25(5 Suppl):S12-7. doi: 10.1016/s0885-3924(03)00065-4. PMID: 12694988.
https://pubmed.ncbi.nlm.nih.gov/12694988/

Hicks CW, Selvin E. Epidemiology of Peripheral Neuropathy and Lower Extremity Disease in Diabetes. Curr Diab Rep. 2019 Aug 27;19(10):86. doi: 10.1007/s11892-019-1212-8. PMID: 31456118; PMCID: PMC6755905.
https://pubmed.ncbi.nlm.nih.gov/31456118/

HPS2-THRIVE Collaborative Group; Landray MJ, Haynes R, Hopewell JC, et al. Effects of extended-release niacin with laropiprant in high-risk patients. N Engl J Med. 2014 Jul 17;371(3):203-12. doi: 10.1056/NEJMoa1300955. PMID: 25014686.
https://pubmed.ncbi.nlm.nih.gov/25014686/

Jeon HS, Kang SY, Park JH, Lee HS. Effects of pulsed electromagnetic field therapy on delayed-onset muscle soreness in biceps brachii. Phys Ther Sport. 2015 Feb;16(1):34-9. doi: 10.1016/j.ptsp.2014.02.006. Epub 2014 Mar 7. PMID: 24906295.
https://pubmed.ncbi.nlm.nih.gov/24906295/

Kessler NJ, Lockard MM, Fischer J. Whole body vibration improves symptoms of diabetic peripheral neuropathy. J Bodyw Mov Ther. 2020 Apr;24(2):1-3. doi: 10.1016/j.jbmt.2020.01.004. Epub 2020 Feb 11. PMID: 32507132. https://pubmed.ncbi.nlm.nih.gov/32507132/

Kharrazian D, Herbert M, Vojdani A. Detection of Islet Cell Immune Reactivity with Low Glycemic Index Foods: Is This a Concern for Type 1 Diabetes? J Diabetes Res. 2017;2017:4124967. doi: 10.1155/2017/4124967. Epub 2017 Jul 27. PMID: 28819632; PMCID: PMC5551512.
https://www.ncbi.nlm.nih.gov/pmc/articles/PMC5551512/

Laakso M, Kuusisto J, Stancakova A, et al. The Metabolic Syndrome in Men study: A resource for studies of metabolic and cardiovascular diseases. J. Lipid Res. 2017;58:481–493. doi: 10.1194/jlr.O072629.
https://pubmed.ncbi.nlm.nih.gov/28119442/

Liu YD, Wang ZB, Han G, Zhao P. Hyperbaric oxygen treatment attenuates neuropathic pain by elevating autophagy flux via inhibiting mTOR pathway. Am J Transl Res. 2017 May 15;9(5):2629-2638. PMID: 28560010; PMCID: PMC5446542.
https://pubmed.ncbi.nlm.nih.gov/28560010/

Min HK, Kim SH, Choi JH, et al. Impacts of statin and metformin on neuropathy in patients with type 2 diabetes

mellitus: Korean Health Insurance data. World J Clin Cases. 2021 Nov 26;9(33):10198-10207. doi: 10.12998/wjcc.v9.i33.10198. PMID: 34904090; PMCID: PMC8638058.
https://www.ncbi.nlm.nih.gov/pmc/articles/PMC863805 8/

Peet M. International variations in the outcome of schizophrenia and the prevalence of depression in relation to national dietary practices: an ecological analysis. Br J Psychiatry. 2004 May;184:404-8. doi: 10.1192/bjp.184.5.404. PMID: 15123503.
https://pubmed.ncbi.nlm.nih.gov/15123503/

Psychology Today, July 24 2022, Depression Is Not Caused By Chemical Imbalance In The Brain, by Norman Spencer, Ph.D.
https://www.psychologytoday.com/intl/blog/insight-therapy/202207/depression-is-not-caused-chemical-imbalance-in-the-brain

Sanchez A, Reeser JL, Lau HS, et al. Role of sugars in human neutrophilic phagocytosis. Am J Clin Nutr. 1973 Nov;26(11):1180-4. doi: 10.1093/ajcn/26.11.1180. PMID: 4748178. https://academic.oup.com/ajcn/article-abstract/26/11/1180/4732762

Schiavo S, DeBacker J, Djaiani C, et al. Mechanistic Rationale and Clinical Efficacy of Hyperbaric Oxygen Therapy in Chronic Neuropathic Pain: An Evidence-Based Narrative Review. Pain Res Manag. 2021 Apr 22;2021:8817504. doi: 10.1155/2021/8817504. PMID: 33976752; PMCID: PMC8084668.
https://pubmed.ncbi.nlm.nih.gov/33976752/

Sperling RI. The effects of dietary n-3 polyunsaturated fatty acids on neutrophils. Proc Nutr Soc. 1998 Nov;57(4):527-34. doi: 10.1079/pns19980077. PMID: 10096112. https://pubmed.ncbi.nlm.nih.gov/10096112/

Tristan Asensi M, Napoletano A, Sofi F, Dinu M. Low-Grade Inflammation and Ultra-Processed Foods Consumption: A Review. Nutrients. 2023 Mar 22;15(6):1546. doi: 10.3390/nu15061546. PMID: 36986276; PMCID: PMC10058108. https://pubmed.ncbi.nlm.nih.gov/36986276/

Walz J, Hinzmann J, Haase I, Witte T. Ganzkörperhyperthermie in der Schmerztherapie. Eine kontrollierte Studie an Patienten mit Fibromyalgiesyndrom [Whole body hyperthermia in pain therapy. A controlled trial on patients with fibromyalgia]. Schmerz. 2013 Feb;27(1):38-45. German. doi: 10.1007/s00482-012-1288-4. PMID: 23354314. https://pubmed.ncbi.nlm.nih.gov/23354314/

Yamany AAM, Bitesha K Effect of 850 nm He-Ne Laser Therapy on Nerve Conduction and Foot Planter Pressures Distribution of Painful Diabetic Neuropathy: A Randomized Controlled Trial. J Nov Physiother. 2016; 6: 300. doi:10.4172/2165-7025.1000300 https://www.omicsonline.org/open-access-pdfs/effect-of-850-nm-hene-laser-therapy-on-nerve-conduction-andfoot-planter-pressures-distribution-of-painful-diabetic-neuropathy-aran-2165-7025-1000300.pdf

Zarief E. Ozone Therapy in Clinical, Psychological and Neurophysiological Pain Alleviation in Patients With Diabetic Neuropathy. Clinical Trial https://clinicaltrials.gov/ct2/show/NCT05000463

Zhao B, Pan Y, Xu H, Song X. Hyperbaric oxygen attenuates neuropathic pain and reverses inflammatory signaling likely via the Kindlin-1/Wnt-10a signaling pathway in the chronic pain injury model in rats. J Headache Pain. 2017 Dec;18(1):1. doi: 10.1186/s10194-016-0713-y. Epub 2017 Jan 5. Erratum in: J Headache Pain. 2022 Mar 4;23(1):32. PMID: 28058534; PMCID: PMC5216011.

https://pubmed.ncbi.nlm.nih.gov/28058534/

RESOURCES

Peripheral Neuropathy Support Groups:

https://www.foundationforpn.org/support/support-groups/

https://neuropathycommons.org/content/neuropathy-support-groups

Peripheral Neuropathy Forums:

https://www.smartpatients.com/communities/peripheral-neuropathy

https://connect.mayoclinic.org/discussion/living-with-neuropathy-welcome-to-the-group/

Facebook Group for Peripheral Neuropathy:

https://www.facebook.com/groups/2874002256011100/

Diabetes Support Groups:

https://defeatdiabetes.org/get-healthy/diabetes-support-groups/

https://professional.diabetes.org/content-page/diabetes-support-directory

https://community.beyondtype2.org/

Made in United States
Troutdale, OR
10/16/2023

13747292R00120